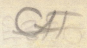

RELATIVE STRANGER

Mary Loudon is also the author of *Secrets and Lives: Middle England Revealed; Revelations: The Clergy Questioned* and *Unveiled: Nuns Talking*. All three were published to enormous critical acclaim.

Mary has won four writing prizes and contributed to four anthologies. She is an experienced broadcaster and critic, has chaired many public discussions and been a Whitbread Prize judge.

She lives in Oxfordshire and the Wye Valley with her husband and children.

Also by Mary Loudon

Secrets and Lives: Middle England Revealed
Revelations: The Clergy Questioned
Unveiled: Nuns Talking

RELATIVE STRANGER

A Sister's Life After Death

MARY LOUDON

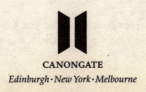

CANONGATE

Edinburgh · New York · Melbourne

First published in Great Britain in 2006 by
Canongate Books Ltd, 14 High Street,
Edinburgh EH1 1TE

This paperback edition first published by Canongate Books Ltd in 2007

1

British Library Cataloguing-in-Publication Data
A catalogue record for this book is available on
request from the British Library

978 1 84195 894 1 (13-digit ISBN)
1 84195 894 8 (10-digit ISBN)

Typeset in Sabon by Palimpsest Book Production Ltd, Grangemouth, Stirlingshire
Printed and bound in Great Britain by Clays Ltd, St Ives plc

www.canongate.net

*Clare, Jane and Celia, my beautiful daughters,
this book is for you*

'Is not the life more than meat, and the body than raiment?'

Matthew, chapter six, verse 25

Contents

PART ONE: END

Same Time, Different Place

On the twenty-seventh of January 2001, while I was skiing fast down a mountain in France, my sister, Catherine, was dying slowly in England; in a hospital I didn't know she had been admitted to, from a cancer I didn't know she had, under an identity I had no idea existed.

Catherine was my eldest sister, the third of five children. I am the fifth and youngest. When she died, she was forty-seven and I was thirty-four.

Born into a well-off family, we five were an undoubtedly privileged lot. On paper, we could look pretty obnoxious. We grew up in a beautiful house with parents who loved us well. We were broadly educated, widely travelled and generally encouraged. When I left home, I had a good life. I went to university, made friends, went to parties, and travelled with a backpack. I began writing books, bought a house and had a fair number of nice boyfriends. Then I married a lovely man and had a baby. Certainly, minor things went wrong from time to time, and I suffered one fairly serious bout of depression in my early twenties, but apart from that I enjoyed great good fortune.

When Catherine left home she went to India for a year where she became seriously ill, suffered the breakdown from which she never fully recovered, and then vanished. After a fraught search by the Foreign Office and our father she was found but vanished for a second time. Some time later, she finally returned home to England, broken.

After that, she went to Oxford, first to a bedsit, then to Oxford prison and then to Oxford's psychiatric hospital, the Warneford. After a brief ensuing stint in Holloway jail and a spell in Guy's hospital, London, she went to live quietly in a council flat in Bristol. There she kept a private home. In the beginning, it was open only to the homeless and the vagrant; in the end, to no one. After she turned twenty she appears to have had no lovers and we, her family, were not encouraged to visit her. There were no holidays, no parties, no steady job and no children. Once, for a time, she owned and loved a dog.

During the last eleven years of Catherine's life, the few requests she made for visits from us were invariably rescinded by her, and we never saw her alive again.

It looks as if Catherine and I began our lives in the same place but we didn't. She had schizophrenia and I did not.

The Sort Of Phone Call Everybody Dreads

My mother was due to visit us at our house in Wales the next day. So when she rang I assumed it was to discuss the usual details like whether she would be bringing her dog, why she wouldn't be driving through the centre of Hereford and what food she was leaving for my father.

Instead, she said, 'I've got some sad news. It's about Catherine.'

'Catherine?'

My mother is a woman who always gets straight to the point.

'Catherine died.'

'Oh, no. Oh, Mummy.'

My husband, Andrew, was at our neighbours' house. I phoned them and asked for him.

'Hey,' he said, 'what's up?'

'Please come home now.'

There was merriment in the background. Andrew was chuckling at something someone was saying. He was distracted.

'What's the problem, darling?'

'It's okay, it's not the baby. My sister's dead. Catherine died.'

Catherine had been admitted to the Bristol Royal Infirmary over Christmas with advanced, inoperable cancer and she had stated, very firmly, that she had no next of kin.

Two parents, four brothers and sisters, each with spouses and children. No next of kin?

So, not surprisingly, the hospital never contacted us, she was forty-seven years old after all, not four; and there she died on 27th January surrounded by no flowers, no grapes, no cards and no relatives, which was clearly exactly what she wanted. Afterwards, the authorities went into her flat. Someone found some unopened post. Someone else opened it and found an address. Someone else put two and two together, although not terribly quickly, and eleven days later a Bristol City Council Registrar telephoned my parents.

Lucky, really. It doesn't have to work out that way. She might have vanished altogether that last time. And there were some mercies, I suppose. At least there was still a body and a body means a funeral. And a funeral means a meeting of sorts, albeit one-sided.

Shock

Think of a wall made of tissue paper and a giant fist punching through it, without warning.

It felt a bit like that, if you can imagine such a thing.

Anger (and not a little admiration)

'No next of kin?' says a close family friend. 'Wow. It might just as well be suicide, as far as the aggression of that denial goes.'

Someone else adds: 'You've got to hand it to her. She always was a stubborn bastard.'

Grief

The world turned dark grey. It didn't help that it was February.

Acceptance

What is there not to accept? You can't rewind a death.

Relief

Relief was almost universally expressed when people outside the family learned that my dead sister was Catherine and not my other sister or me. Gratitude was expressed too, when people learnt that she had died of natural causes. Everybody thinks that schizophrenics commit suicide, if they don't kill other people.

Some Things People Said When They Found Out

A neighbour: 'You should look at it this way. At least you won't have to look after her when she's old.'

An old boyfriend: 'Darling, I'm so sorry, it's absolutely terrible, but you know what? Some people are made for this world, some people aren't.'

A family friend: 'At least it was only cancer. Just think how much worse it could have been with her being – well, you know.'

Various others: 'Thank God she didn't commit suicide.'
  'At least she's in peace now.'
  'It must be a merciful release in a way.'
  'Well, you weren't really that close to her, were you.'
  'How terrible for your parents. But it's better in a way they know what's happened to her, than that they die wondering.'
  'Oh, I'm terribly sorry. I thought she was dead already.'

Dreams and Nightmares

When someone is asleep and they cannot tell the difference between what is real and what is imaginary, they are dreaming.

When someone is awake and they cannot tell the difference between what is real and what is imaginary, they are having a nightmare, from which even sleep is no escape. This nightmare is commonly described as a 'psychotic illness'.

The most common of these psychotic illnesses is schizophrenia. Schizophrenia does not mean, and has never meant, 'split personality'. Schizophrenia means 'divided mind' and is a direct reference to the splitting or fragmentation of an individual's thinking and feeling processes, a symptom which is typical of and central to the illness.

Schizophrenia is global and cross-cultural. It has no definite known cause although there are a number of possible causal factors involved in its onset and development, and while some of its symptoms are treatable it is as yet incurable.

Much of what we assume about schizophrenia is not true. Contrary to popular belief schizophrenics are statistically no more violent than the rest of the population. A diagnosis of major mental illness is far less predictive of violence than being young, male, single, and under the influence of alcohol. Consider your average Saturday-night drunk, released at closing time from the pub into the community, unfocused and aggressive, his own mental disorder absolutely in place.

Another common misconception is that most schizo-phrenics commit suicide. Around 10% of schizophrenics commit suicide. This is ten times higher than the figure for the general population but it still leaves 90% of schizo-phrenics to die like other people.

The symptoms of schizophrenia fall into two categories, positive and negative. Positive symptoms create sensations when there is nothing there to be sensed, or the generation of thought patterns that the sufferer can't control. These are often accompanied by bizarre beliefs, such as being God. Negative symptoms feature the reduction or even oblitera-tion of normal mental or behavioural processes.

Some positive symptoms include:

auditory hallucinations: hearing things that are not there, often voices.

delusions: a belief in thought insertion (the sufferer is convinced that outsiders are inserting or tampering with thoughts), thought withdrawal (the removal of thoughts by a third party which leaves the mind 'blank'), or thought broadcasting (when a hostile outside force causes thoughts to be heard by others).

thought disorder and speech abnormalities: the sufferer makes muddled and illogical conversation, often with surreal results. Relationships between ideas are disjointed or non-existent and associations are loosened. Sometimes the sufferer jumps ahead of him- or herself in conversation, or 'talks past the point', producing rambling and complex responses even to simple yes/no questions.

other hallucinations: visual (seeing things that are not there), olfactory (smelling things that are not there), gustatory (tasting something non-existent) and somatic (the experi-encing of persistent pains).

Some negative symptoms include:

emotional blunting: an impaired ability to express emotion by verbal or non-verbal means. This is not a matter of choice: the sufferer simply doesn't possess the expressive capacity of the ordinary individual. In some cases, he or she doesn't even experience the internal sensation of an emotion.

poverty of speech and speech content: the sufferer says little and rarely initiates conversation. Speech may convey little or no meaning or it may stop and restart after long intervals.

avolition: a lack of will to act at all.

anhedonia: the inability to experience pleasure to a normal degree.

asociality: the avoidance of the company of others. The asocial sufferer may have no friends at all but not regard this as a problem. He or she may also have no romantic or sexual interest whatever.

Schizophrenics tend to suffer either positive or negative symptoms, although some may experience symptoms from each category. But either broad set of symptoms confers upon sufferers a terrible sentence: vivid, surround-sound nightmares or life with all the colour removed.

My sister, Catherine, heard voices.

She saw people who weren't there.

She believed that MI5 and the Police were following her.

She thought there were people inside her head, telling her what to do.

She exhibited odd and disturbing behaviour. She would grin and laugh for no apparent reason and rock herself backwards and forwards. She would prowl the house at 3 a.m. or visit the local police station to discuss the Dalai Lama. A few times, she took off her clothes in the street.

She found it difficult to maintain a conversation on one subject for more than a minute or two.

She told lies, not all of which she necessarily believed.

For some years, she was frequently aggressive and hostile.

She was unable to hold down a job.

She could not maintain relationships that demanded anything of her.

Occasionally, she experienced moments of total lucidity, which appeared to cause her great joy or profound pain.

From around the age of twenty-one she could not sleep in the dark.

When she was a teenager my sister took drugs. She began with nicotine, no doubt smoking behind the proverbial bike shed at school from an alarmingly early age. It certainly wasn't allowed at home.

She progressed to cannabis, with a group of her friends, which earned them all expulsion from their smart girls' school. When she left home, and later travelled overseas, she found all sorts of other drugs to try as well.

Whether or not the drugs caused her most catastrophic breakdowns is unclear. Psychologically speaking, she was by no means at home within herself from very early childhood. That she was mentally vulnerable was certain. But the causal factors implicated in schizophrenia, whether they are hereditary, genetic or chemical (and it is most likely they are a highly complex combination of all three) are so various that it is impossible to be sure how the illness is produced in each individual, and whether or not its onset could have been avoided.

However, this much is known:

The majority of psycho-mimetic and psychedelic drugs, such as LSD, are believed capable of triggering schizophrenia in some people.

The use of powerful psychedelics can also cause a range of symptoms resembling those produced by schizophrenia.

Recent research suggests that the same may be true of cannabis, if used excessively.

Stimulants, such as amphetamine (speed) and cocaine, are also capable of producing forms of psychosis. Long-term use of cocaine is often associated with delusions of persecution.

Ecstasy is believed to cause schizophrenia-like symptoms to develop in some people.

Around the world, Stone Age skulls have been discovered with holes made in them. Evidence of bone re-growth shows that these holes were made when the person was alive. It is believed that the holes were made to provide a portal from which evil spirits could escape, spirits that the poor soul whose skull was being hammered or drilled was assumed to be harbouring.

Supernatural explanations remained the dominant theory behind mental illness for centuries so that until recently, if you were crazy, the chances are that you were regarded as being possessed either by the divine or the devil. It's quite a thought, really, that the early Christian saints, with their visions and their voices from on high, were very possibly suffering from schizophrenic delusions and hallucinations. That, plus dehydration and sunstroke. It's also sobering to recall that, fifteen centuries later, those women possessed of similar visions and voices were burnt at the stake as witches. (Although, if the Virgin Mary made an appearance in any of these visions, increasingly the possessed were rewarded with sanctification and the Virgin with a shrine.)

My medieval sister would most likely have ended up on the stake or, if she'd been born a couple of centuries later, in a straitjacket or chains. Of course, there was always the street, a space occupied by members of the schizophrenic population still. So it's lucky she was born into an age and culture of relative enlightenment. She had electro-convulsive therapy, anti-psychotic drugs and other people's ignorance and non-specific fears to contend with. Admittedly, they're not a great list but they have to be better than a fire or shackles.

For those unfortunate enough to develop schizophrenia the road ahead is long and uncertain. The chance of remaining symptomatic and needing long-term, high levels of social and medical input after a single episode of schizophrenia is twenty per cent. The chance of a partial recovery after a single episode of schizophrenia is sixty per cent. The chance of a full recovery after a single episode of schizophrenia is only twenty per cent, which means that if you develop schizophrenia the odds are eight out of ten that you will never be rid of it.

Parents and siblings of schizophrenics are on average ten times more likely to develop the condition themselves than members of the general population. Children of schizophrenics are nearly fifteen times more likely to develop the condition and identical twins of schizophrenics forty-seven times more likely.

The average risk is one in a hundred and it may not sound like a lot. But if you think of everyone you know the chances are that some of them, or their immediate family members, are schizophrenics. We don't discuss it a lot, this kind of reality. We don't even give it much thought. Instead, our abstract fears tend to be about disasters we imagine may befall us even though the risk of their doing so is very low, like plane crashes. One way of putting such morbid fantasies into perspective is to visit the web-site of the Office for National Statistics and do some sums. Then, you can work out that you are more likely – assuming you buy the relevant tickets – to win the National Lottery than to plummet from the sky in an aeroplane. And you are twenty times more likely to develop schizophrenia in your lifetime than to die or be seriously injured in a road traffic accident.

Words and Pictures

The night I heard about her death I went through Catherine's letters.

Though I lingered it needn't have taken long. There weren't many of them, for a start; one a year, if that, over the last fifteen years and they were mostly fairly short. Her writing was pretty poor, it was scrawly. She wrote on an upwards diagonal with a lot of space around each word and each line, and within each word every letter stood alone. It seemed that her handwriting grew perfectly to reflect the solitary, isolated personality that she was. In her early letters it was neater, flowing, straightforward. In her later ones, it was utterly disjointed. The letters were also full of slang: 'cos' for 'because', 'ain't' for 'isn't', 'jis' for 'just'.

And I considered what it was to write to someone.

Writing to her I thought was enough. There was Christmas and her birthday. On top, I'd write maybe six times a year. I'd send photos, sometimes phone cards and money. I wasn't brilliant but I kept in touch and while the letters from her average out at one a year for the last fifteen years of her life, some years there were none. Sometimes, I could go for months and months writing into a void so profound that I believed she would never again emerge from it. There would be absolute silence and then, out of the blue, a letter, or occasionally, a phone call. The last one of those was in 1995.

When I was a small child there were lots of letters. When I was a teenager there were dozens of phone calls. She would phone home high and angry or wildly enthusiastic about something. The calls were always disturbing because her speech was so rapid and slurred with mania that it was difficult to understand what she was saying. In fact, I think she only ever considered the phone as a means of communication when she was at her most manic.

The subjects of the calls were pretty similar. MI5 was after her. She prayed to the Buddha – did I? She needed to see the Dalai Lama because there was so much trouble in Tibet. Sometimes she said she actually was the Dalai Lama. She wanted to know what I thought of the Pope. Could I send her a fiver? And there were often voices, none in particular, just 'they', that she described to me and about which I was totally confused. Almost nothing she said in those phone calls made sense although I got the impression, over the years, that 'they' had stopped asking her to do things. Instead, 'they' just informed on the people who were after her, because as far as she was concerned someone usually was.

So I wrote to her. I listened when she phoned and sometimes but by no means always sent the money that she asked for. I never visited her because she didn't want me to. I never arrived unsolicited at her flat although many times I thought about it. When I considered heading to Bristol armed with groceries I always ended up deciding, correctly, that I had absolutely no right to do so. So I wrote.

But as for reading her letters, that was something I clearly hadn't done all that well. For reading them that night, knowing her gone for ever, I was consumed with regret, overwhelmed with the feeling that I'd missed what was there when I had the chance to respond to it properly. I was busy, I was wrapped up in my own life: writing books, falling in love, moving house, having a baby, whatever. In her last letter to me she wrote, *I'm in bad health but in fine spirits.*

She was upbeat. She said how lucky Andrew and I were to have a house in the Wye Valley and how much she liked the look of it (I'd sent her a picture). I remember writing back, concerned about her health, offering to help in any way she wanted. She didn't reply. I know now that she was afraid she was dying.

With her letters in my lap, I sat on the cream sofa in my white study, with its cream rug and its soft light, and its muted watercolours and black and white photographs on the wall. I sat in the harmony I had so carefully created and in my sister's scrawl saw my own flaw writ large. I re-read the letters, some written on yellowish scraps of spiral-bound notepaper, and they informed me anew that I'd missed my sister while she was here and now it was too late. I had failed to perceive the sort of person she was from those letters. The letters had jokes in them and funny stories. I simply hadn't realised. I hadn't seen them at the time. Why didn't I see that she liked jokes? They were pretty crummy jokes, admittedly, Christmas cracker jokes in fact, but still jokes. How did I fail to notice that she liked funny stories? Why didn't I write back with my jokes and my funny stories? Oh, I always wrote back straightaway, the good sister that I was. The stupid damned sister, as it turns out. Frightened of Catherine's idiosyncrasies, I sent her cheerful, nothingy post cards or short newsy letters containing no information that could threaten, harm or be misconstrued. They were supposed to be soothing. How anodyne they must have been, each and every one. How disappointing.

How easy it is to let fear banish good sense and clear vision and to fall into the trap of thinking that for the mentally ill even the barest contact is enough and that scraps of information, rather than nourishing communication, will suffice. You see this sort of thing all the time in homes for the elderly: 'Hello dear, and how are we this morning? Ready for breakfast? Rise and shine.' That's a bit of a cliché but we all get entrapped by clichés at some time or another. We seek refuge in banalities when afraid. People did it to me when Catherine died. Did I do it to her when she was alive?

When Catherine was alive, all I ever read in her letters was deterioration. All I saw was hard evidence of her disintegration. This wasn't just because I compared the letters with the level of communication and responsiveness that had gone before. It was because I compared them with what I imagined might have been. I contrasted them with the sort of person I thought she could have become. I realise now how fatuous such thoughts were because the person Catherine could have become, she became. Schizophrenia wasn't a car accident that happened to her when she was eighteen. It didn't put her in a metaphorical wheelchair and cut off her brilliant life, although that doesn't stop people seeing it that way. Schizophrenia didn't arrive and suddenly remove her faculties because schizophrenia was already part of them, already built in. It came with her. It was part of the whole package. Catherine was never going to be anyone else. She was never going to develop differently, or not in any significant way.

There seems to me now no question that Catherine's deterioration was an integral part of her developing self and no doubt that her illness was not so much a process of fragmentation but a progress. However, because development is associated with complexity as opposed to simplification, and progress with unity, not division, they are not the sorts of words usually used to describe the effect on a person of the relentless advance of schizophrenia.

Trying to see a person through the fog of serious mental illness is a little bit like trying to make sense of someone speaking to you in a language of which you have only a basic grasp. You do a lot of filling in. You nod and smile

and agree and hope that you are stumbling along the right
track whilst suspecting, often correctly, that you are nowhere
near it. Sometimes, you find that you are completely lost. I
found this with Catherine. Over the years, she sent me quite
a lot of presents and they invariably made me sad. They
were so poignant, or at least that's what I felt. She sent a
long necklace, its mock-seed beads bright turquoise and red,
childish in style – or so I thought at the time. Gently fingering
it that night in my study, admiring its delicacy, I could not
understand why I had misconstrued it so. She sent a small
plastic key for good luck when Andrew and I were engaged.
She sent a very nice pair of pyjamas the Christmas after we
were married: *You can fight over who wears which half*, she
wrote. I remember being deeply touched when I received the
key. I was struck by the gentle, old-fashioned convention-
ality of the gesture, coming as it did from one of the least
conventional people I have ever known. However, if my old
school-friend Joe, who loves kitsch, had sent me that key I'd
have received it quite differently. It would have made me
smile. I would have recognised and appreciated the irony in
it, had it come from someone not remotely convinced by the
mores of betrothal. It is Joe's instinct to respond to something he regards as bourgeois by taking the mick. From
Catherine, the key was confusing.

There was something about Catherine's presents that hurt
me. I think it's because I didn't understand them, by which
I mean they had no solid context for me. I have a Godmother
who sends me pretty tea towels and my knowledge of her
means that the tea towels make sense. I know they're the
kind of thing she likes herself and I know they represent also
the way she sees me now, as a mother at home with children and the washing-up. But Catherine's presents never did
make sense, or not entirely, because I didn't know enough
any more. I didn't really know quite who she was, so how

could I understand what her presents meant? On the other hand, because I knew she was ill, odd, weird, I was always a little alarmed by them. So I filled in for myself the bits I didn't understand. I did a lot of guessing, just as you do with the foreign language in which you are not proficient. I nodded and smiled, understanding the necessary minimum, whilst feeling perplexed.

It is said that a little learning is a dangerous thing and maybe that's what it was. Knowing that Catherine was ill is my justification, my explanation, for my fear of her and her presents. Fair enough, I suppose, but perhaps Catherine felt exactly about the world the way I did about her communications with me. Perhaps, for her, the world was all information without context, like noise without an obvious source. Perhaps the world itself was a foreign language, full of its own strange and brutal grammar. Perhaps it was never a relatively straightforward environment but instead a place of unfathomable unreliability, filled with disembodied voices and unexpected, and therefore unsettling, intrusions.

With a schizophrenic you're always trying to read between the lines. You're always trying to make sense of the confusion with which you're presented. Maybe it cuts both ways. Maybe that's exactly what the paranoia that Catherine was diagnosed with feels like. Maybe being paranoid is routinely to assume that something is more than it is. Catherine sent me a necklace and a necklace is just a necklace. If it means anything at all, it means, Wear me, decorate yourself, you'll look good. I see now that in this particular instance Catherine understood that and I didn't. I was seeing things in that necklace that were not there. If that's the case, what did my failure to accept her gifts for what they were imply about my acceptance of her? Why could I not take them simply at face value, the way one might accept a compliment or good wish from a relative stranger? Is it because she wasn't a relative stranger or because, in fact, that's precisely what she was?

Catherine also sent me a lot of her paintings. She had always drawn and painted and was unquestionably good enough to become an artist or illustrator. Our father has always had a parallel career to medicine and writing as an artist and if such talent is inherited then Catherine inherited his. As a child and teenager she could work in any medium, and did so. Oils, watercolour, pen and ink, pencil. She was capable of ferocity in her work: covering one entire side of her bedroom door at home was a deep, dark forest, in vivid midnight blues and greens. One of the trees in the foreground doubled up as a naked woman, dark blue and greeny white, with tendrils for hair. In art-history terms, it looked a bit Dali-esque and a bit pre-Raphaelite, with a touch of Arthur Rackham. That makes it sound like a dog's breakfast but it wasn't. It was disturbing and fabulous.

She was also capable of great tenderness. In contrast to her huge oils were perfect and tiny (envelope-sized) pencil drawings of the family and our dogs and cats. She wrote and illustrated two books for me. I read them now to my daughters, marvelling at the gorgeous, melancholic animals. Her watercolours were delicate and exquisite and in all her pictures - landscapes, animals and figures – there was something beautiful but troubling. They accommodated a lot of her sadness, fear and anger. It was as if in her pictures she was expressing and responding to everything that was alien to her in the things that she saw and the people she knew.

Years after these subtly refined paintings and drawings were done, what I received through the post from Catherine were luridly coloured, two-dimensional paintings of parrots, jays, tigers, Tibetan warriors and Hindu temples. All of them had heavy outlines, with black lines marking clearly delineated sections of wing, jaw, sword or minaret. Each section was coloured in with care. No two sections overlapped.

There was no mixing of colours, no grey areas. The most extraordinary feature of these pictures was that while each one was clearly a work of the imagination none of them looked original. They all looked as if they had been copied or traced.

I've since learned from psychiatrists who work with people like my sister that these characteristics are typically found in pictures done by those who suffer from schizophrenia or autism. This fact made me feel better for a while and then worse. It was as if the pictures' lack of originality further emphasised just how great was the depredation of Catherine's personality by her ravaging illness.

The artist Catherine became would neither have made a living from her work nor achieved Sunday-newspaper recognition, or illustrated children's books. The artist she became was prolific and dedicated, obsessive even, while the art itself was cruder, imitative, repetitive. Many people would say that her paintings were childish. Some might say that a child could have done them. In fact, few children could, for their lack of innocence was one of their most striking features. But does it matter what they looked like? I'm not sure what makes an artist, after all. The quality of the work or the impulse, necessity even, to produce it?

'It's a shame,' said a friend, 'that she never realised her potential. She was so incredibly talented. She could easily have made a good living as an artist.'

I don't blame my friend for thinking that way. I used to. Over time, though, I came to see that Catherine did realise her potential as an artist. If there was any failure of realisation it was ours, which I don't think surprising, and I don't think it is anything to be ashamed of, either. After all, you have to take a huge step away from inculcated views about progress in order to understand that a person's potential may still be fulfilled even if its expression becomes cruder, not subtler; even if her pictures are more colourful and less delicate, more simplistic and less mature. However, as long as realisation of potential is confused with betterment the general supposition will remain that fulfilment of promise is dependent upon technical improvement and not, instead, on the capacity of a human being to engage with the world and produce a response to it.

The evolution of a human individual is anything but straightforward. If Darwin's survival theory had been applied to Catherine's evolution as an artist today there is no doubt that she would have perished, for her work would have been deemed unfit for exhibition. But that's only if you believe that to be an artist is to be recognised as such by others besides you. As it happens, Catherine's work was recognised by others. Not only did she give it away to people she knew, she organised an exhibition in a local café where her pictures were displayed willingly and for some time. I know that Catherine was proud of what she did and I know she spent hours doing it. I know that painting brought her joy because she wrote about it often, in her letters to me. She told people she was an artist and I know she knew that's who and what she was. What I'll never know is whether she remembered her earlier work – work that was deemed by others to be promising, exciting and beautiful – and whether, if she did, she considered it at all in relation to her later output. I doubt it even matters.

Of one thing I am sure. Schizophrenia destroyed, reduced and corrupted aspects of Catherine's personality in all sorts of ways, and nothing has led me to believe that there was anything romantic or lovely about the process. But that night, curled up way past midnight on my cream sofa, tears streaming down my face, something more than Catherine was revealed to me as her words and pictures swam before me. I began to see that progress and reduction are not mutually exclusive and that the thing we call potential is complicated by the human organism in which it develops. I began to realise that a woman who reaches her potential may yet be one of the most broken examples of humanity that we – those others who consider ourselves more or less whole – know how to describe.

Visit To the Morgue

My realisation that I wanted badly to see my sister's body came pretty late. It was Friday afternoon and the funeral was scheduled for the following Wednesday. Suddenly panicky at the thought that I might miss her this final time, I telephoned the Bristol Royal Infirmary at five o'clock, which is not an ideal time to call anyone.

I was put through to the mortuary by the switchboard operator but there was no reply.

'I think they've all gone home,' she said. 'You'll need to call back on Monday and ask to arrange a time to view a patient.'

So you're a patient as long as you're in the hospital, even if you're dead. Presumably only when you are released for disposal are you a proper corpse.

'Okay,' I said, 'thank you. I will.'

'And you'll need the patient's hospital number,' said the switchboard operator.

'Right.'

'Have you got that?'

'Yes, I've got it.'

Monday. I rang the mortuary again.

Catherine's hospital number was BRI 663909 and only when I looked at it that day did I feel that she was really dead. Often, the departed feel only partially absent to the recently bereaved because the fact of their departure simply hasn't sunk in. But now, the statistical impersonality of Catherine's hospital number confirmed to me that she was finished, despite the fact that it was originally assigned to her living, breathing version.

'Hello,' said the mortuary technician. 'Mr Carpenter speaking.'

I explained who I was and that I wanted to come and see my sister.

I said, 'I have her hospital number.'

'It's all right, Mrs St George,' he said, using my married name and not the name by which I was related to the body in his care, 'I won't need that. Normally, viewing times are between two and four in the afternoon but if it's better for you, coming so far with a baby and everything, you can come at midday.'

I was grateful. I didn't want to view her body in the afternoon. It was truly vile outside, pouring with rain, and the forecast was the same for the following day. The thought of going to see her at the dog end of a February day, in the wet and dark after driving around Bristol in busy traffic, was awful.

I was about to say to him, 'I don't actually want to see her face, I just want to hold her hand,' but he pre-empted me.

He said, 'You won't be able to see the body, I'm afraid. It'll be covered up and you won't be able to see it uncovered because the deceased is not in a very good state.'

The deceased. All these terms we attach to various rites of passage. Bride and groom, new Mum, pensioner, the deceased. And it doesn't matter who you are, or how old, if you end up in a mortuary you're 'the deceased', referred to no longer by name, title or occupation but state. I don't suppose there's any way around that one, no way around the fact that had Mr Carpenter been discussing someone else's relative there would have been nothing to differentiate between that person and Catherine.

'It's okay,' I replied. 'I don't want to see her face or anything, I just want . . . Under a cloth is fine. I just want to touch her body.'

'That's fine,' said Mr Carpenter, 'we'll arrange that.'

Tuesday.

The entrance to the mortuary of the Bristol Royal Infirmary was on Lower Maudlin Street. On a different day, I might have smiled. The street was short, narrow and quite steep, with the mortuary halfway down it through some heavy Victorian iron gates. There was an electric car barrier beyond the gates, and beyond the barrier some double doors that looked like an old-fashioned tradesmen's entrance. I was to ring the bell at the doors and somebody would come. In the event, there was no need because three people were standing in front of the doors, one of whom I recognised immediately as Mr Carpenter. Fiftyish, solid, his arms folded over a thick, wool jersey, it was evidently him because he was the only man obviously waiting for someone.

'Mr Carpenter?'

He gestured with his arm towards a side door and the two other men dissolved immediately without my noticing, in the way that people and objects do when obliterated by grief's narrowed vision.

'Hello.' He shook my hand. 'Come this way.'

Turning left, we entered a small, airless foyer. Over-warm and thickly carpeted, it was furnished with a wicker sofa and cushions, two wicker chairs and a side table. On the side table was a square box of tissues and a bowl of dried flowers. The place was like a lobby to a middle-range bed and breakfast.

'Take a seat,' said Mr Carpenter.

Relieved, I sat.

'Please,' I asked, 'before we go in, can we just talk in here? I don't want to go in yet.'

'Is your husband joining you?'

'No. He's in a café around the corner with our daughter. I wanted to do this on my own.'

'Of course.'

Mr Carpenter explained that he could sit quietly in the room with me if I wanted him to. I did want him to. I was frightened. He explained to me that the body was now frozen. The deceased had been dead too long to remain in the refrigerator where a certain amount of decomposition had already taken place, and consequently had had to be put in a freezer. He was sorry about that. I told him that was okay but I had some questions.

I asked him, 'Will she smell? Will she smell of formaldehyde?'

She wouldn't smell.

I asked him how she was covered. In my imagination, I saw a horizontal body's delicate profile beneath a thin white sheet.

She was in a shroud, wrapped in a sheet and two body-bags, with a cloth on top. The body was on a trolley.

Mr Carpenter began to apologise again. He was sorry because normally they prepared bodies and there was a cloth up to the neck, and you could see the face. The deceased in this case was not in a good enough state for them to have done that but there were other things they could have done.

I said I knew that and it was fine. He'd already been exceptionally helpful.

But he was a conscientious man. He didn't want me to feel he was letting me down.

'If we'd had more warning,' he said, 'if we'd known and had more time, we could have prepared her.'

I said, 'I only want to hold her hand.'

'But we could have prepared her for you to do that, if we'd known. We could have thawed her hand.'

I said, 'It doesn't matter, I'll hold it through the cloth.'

Catherine's body was in a small room just off the foyer. The door was at one end of it and once inside the room you had to turn ninety degrees to see the deceased person you had come to visit. I wondered straightaway whether that was deliberate, whether an architect had gone to the trouble of designing the room so that you didn't face the unknown as soon as you entered, or whether it was unplanned. I began to think how interesting it would be to be a hospital architect.

There were no windows in the room and the light was soft, low and orange. Catherine was on a trolley but there would have been no way of knowing that it was a trolley. It looked more like an altar, wide and substantial, an impression created by its being covered with an enormous orange cloth. Before British Rail was sold off and the rolling stock revamped inside, there used to be bright orange curtains on the high-speed trains out of London Paddington. The cloth covering the trolley looked just like those curtains, only heavier.

Catherine's body was also covered, with a piece of yellow material of similar style and weight. Underneath, there was a vague mound. Later, I said to Mr Carpenter, 'I've been watching too many films. I'd expected a white sheet.' I'd expected to be able to see a nose, a mouth, forehead, shoulders, everything, but I couldn't. It was impossible even to make out precisely where Catherine's head was, there was so much bulky padding at the upper end of her body. I could barely determine where her feet were, either.

I stood beside her. I patted her tentatively. She was rock-hard. There was the merest crackle of plastic body-bag.

'Where's her hand?' I asked.

Mr Carpenter emerged from the shadows at the end of the room. He stood next to me and rummaged gently downwards through the orange cloth. Very softly, he patted it. I pressed down on it with my own hand and felt only a hard surface beneath. It could have been anything. I curled my fingers a little. There was a bit of shape there. A little bolder, I moved up her body and stroked her shoulders lightly with the palms of my hands. I wanted very much not to invade her. I walked the length of her body and found what I thought were her feet though I couldn't be sure.

I said to Mr Carpenter, 'It doesn't look like a body. I can't find her. I don't know where she is.'

He replied, 'She's pretty well wrapped. We've done our best to tuck the bags under but it's not very easy.'

He stepped towards Catherine's body and tucked and stuffed the bags quite vigorously underneath it, like someone making a bed. He was deft and efficient. At last, her shape began to emerge, nothing like as clearly as I had imagined it would, but enough to know that it was human.

Mr Carpenter placed his hands gently and firmly on the body.

'Here's her head.

'Here are the shoulders.

'Here are her hands, they're resting on her thighs.

'Here are the feet.'

I walked around the body and held Catherine's other hand. It was more obviously a hand than the first one. I could feel the shape of it resting on her thigh, I could make out the fingers and thumb. I ran my own hand across her stomach. Catherine was always very thin but now she was vast in the middle. I knew she'd had steroids and that she'd puffed up with them, as people do. But she'd also had a secondary tumour in the liver that had swollen to grotesque proportions. It felt like a football and was as large as one.

I grew bolder with my touch and what was left of my sister became familiar enough to me that I was no longer fearful. I talked to her for a few minutes while Mr Carpenter waited silently at the end of the room, his hands clasped loosely before him, his head slightly bowed.

I've often heard people talk about how peaceful it is, being in the presence of the dead, and I've always wondered, Is it really peaceful or is it just that they're dead? Now, I understand. Catherine was pacific in a way that I'd never known her alive. It wasn't because she was frozen solid. It wasn't because I had any sense of her being somewhere better in death than she had been in life. It wasn't because I believed that her spirit was distinct from the indistinct bulk before me and had been freed from it. And it wasn't because the room was almost silent. In fact, the room didn't feel silent. It felt positively animated by peace. There was vitality to the calm that lent it vibrancy, like the very best moments spent quietly in the dead of night with someone alive.

I knew one thing with complete certainty and I cannot explain it. I knew that Catherine was okay.

With my hand on my sister's, I talked easily with Mr Carpenter. I told him a bit about her, about her illness and the fact that we'd not had as much contact with her as we'd have liked. He said, 'I'm one of five. You grow up as a family and then when everybody's grown up they go their own way.'

'Yeah, that's right.'

'And it doesn't always work out for everyone.'

'No.'

He said, 'It's normal. It's what happens.'

Cancer Ward

It was not enough to be with her, dead. I needed to see where she had died.

Mr Carpenter phoned through to Oncology.

I said, 'But I haven't made an appointment. Won't they mind?'

They didn't. Nice of them.

Mr Carpenter said, 'Let me walk you up through the hospital, save you going round the outside of the building and getting wet.'

Kind, good man, Mr Carpenter, with his straightforward manner and woolly jersey. He looked tired and rubbed absentmindedly at his left shoulder with his right hand.

'Hazard of the job,' I remarked.

He agreed.

'I've got a bad shoulder at the moment,' I said. 'I've had it since I heard about Catherine. I think it's mostly psychosomatic, although it's probably also lifting a lively baby.'

I thought about what Mr Carpenter did all week.

I said, 'I expect lifting dead adults is worse.'

Mr Carpenter smiled and continued to rub his shoulder all the way to Oncology.

We chatted amiably.

'Do you ever get people who don't want to leave their relations down there?' I asked him. 'Who find it hard to say goodbye?'

'We had someone once,' he replied, 'where we had to go

to court in the end. They kept coming back to visit their partner. Terrible case. This person wouldn't let us release the body for the funeral. They came back week after week. In the end, we had to tell them they couldn't see the body, it was too badly decomposed. There's a limit to how often you can take someone in and out of the freezer.'

Our route along the corridors of the Bristol Royal Infirmary, many of them underground, was labyrinthine. Oncology was about half a mile from the mortuary and we passed a lot of people on the way: people being wheeled in wheelchairs and rolled in beds; people with drips; people on crutches. In the lift to Oncology were people without their hair.

I don't know when I've ever felt more alive than I did during that walk. I strode those hospital corridors awash with the sick aware of every healthy muscle in my legs and arms, every easy-moving bone in my body. I don't know when I've felt more grateful for the fact that death had not yet caught up with me. Catherine had been dead for two weeks and two days. She'd been refrigerated for nearly a fortnight, frozen for three days. My own vitality was intensified by comparison, my body so quick and warm, hers so stiff and cold. If I had just skiied down a mountain, or walked up one, I could not have felt physically more exhilarated.

Relief at having been with Catherine surged through me. I'd felt as close to her that morning as I had in a very long time. Given that I had not touched her, alive, for thirteen years, touching her dead was suffused with a heightened, and very possibly unreal, sense of connection with her. I wondered, too, whether she might not think – could she do so – that I was taking advantage of her state by being close to her in a way that she did not invite when she was alive. I'd held her hand, cupped her feet in my hands, stroked her forehead as I stroke the foreheads of my children. All these things I would so much have liked to do for her when she was alive and ill and I had to accept that she might have found too great the liberty I took now.

Yet I was the child she sought in the middle of her restive adolescent nights and took to her bed for comfort. In her later, absentee years, she wrote several times to me of her adoration of the baby she still partly believed I was. I know she loved me dearly, so truly I don't think she'd have minded my post-mortem intimacy with her. She knew I had loved her, too.

Mr Carpenter left me at Oncology. Reception was pretty busy, there were a lot of people around, and I waited. I was still worried about turning up virtually unannounced. A big bunch of flowers on the reception desk had a card tucked inside the blooms: it read, 'For Al'.

A nurse turned to me.

'Can I help you?'

I said, 'I'm Mary St George, my maiden name is Loudon. I'm the sister of Catherine Loudon, who died on this ward.'

'Oh yes,' she replied, straightaway. 'Yes. I know.'

'I hope you don't mind me coming. I just wanted to come up and see where she'd been and maybe talk to anyone who knew her, if that's possible. But if I'm in the way, or this is a bad time, please say.'

'No, it isn't at all.'

'Before we go any further,' I said, 'I want you to know that I haven't come to intrude on Catherine. But I also want you to know that she did have next of kin. There are lots of us. My parents are alive, there are four brothers and sisters, we're all married with children and we all cared about her. We would have been here if we'd known, if she'd wanted.'

'I understand,' she said. 'Look, shall we go somewhere quiet?'

In a side room furnished with low, hessian-covered chairs, and tables stacked with dog-eared copies of *Reader's Digest*, I asked the nurse, whose name was Clare, some questions about my sister.

'Let me go and get Jo,' she said. 'Jo's here on duty today and she nursed her a lot. I'll go and see if she's around.'

I picked up the magazine on the table next to the chair. It was a copy of *Majesty* and it was dated 1986. Fifteen years old. Quite some vintage, even for a waiting-room. Prince Andrew was on the cover, looking self-satisfied and overfed. I flicked through it, aimlessly, it was the first thing to hand. I took nothing in. Clare returned to the room with Jo, who began talking rapidly the second she entered it.

'I don't want you to worry,' she said, without introduction. 'He was quite peaceful at the end. He was very private, he . . .'

And she continued but I didn't hear. She had the wrong patient. All I could think was, How embarrassing for her, for me, for all of us in here right now. She thinks she's come in to talk about someone else and she's going to have to say, 'Oh no, I'm really sorry. You're Cathy Loudon's sister,' and then she's going to have to start all over again. For some reason, I found this excruciating.

I must have looked as if I did, too, for she suddenly paused and corrected herself.

She said, 'Oh God, I'm sorry. She.'

'Sorry?'

'She, not he.'

'I'm not with you.'

'I'm sorry, but we knew your sister as Stevie.'

Stevie.

'She was very insistent that she was a man,' said Jo. 'I'm really sorry, is this a shock?'

She turned to Clare.

'I mean, we got so used to him, didn't we, all of us, that we never thought of him as her. We just thought of him as Stevie. That's just who he was to us. He was a real character.'

Stevie.

Well, why not? It hadn't exactly been a typical day so far.

I said, 'Sure. That's okay.'

Jo nodded gratefully.

I couldn't stop myself double-checking, though.

'So you knew her as Stevie?'

'Yes.'

'You knew Stevie as a man, not a woman, right?'

'Yes.'

'That's fine,' I said, stupefied by how calm I felt. 'I don't have a problem with that. I mean, I'm not completely surprised, she was never comfortable with herself, but I can't think of her as anything except Catherine. So while we talk,' and I heard the apology in my voice, 'if I call her Catherine, I hope you won't mind.'

What an extraordinary situation to be in, apologising for calling your sister by her name. Yet it wasn't really her name at the end. If 'Catherine' wasn't what she wanted and wasn't how she saw herself, I guess at some level it's not who she was.

'He was very peaceful,' said Jo. 'I wouldn't want you to worry or think he was in pain. He wasn't. He was very quiet, he kept himself to himself, but he was very peaceful, very calm.'

I asked, 'Did Stevie say he had no next of kin or that he didn't want his family contacted?'

'He said he had no next of kin.'

I half laughed, half choked.

'That's so funny,' I exclaimed. 'I mean, that's such bollocks. There are loads of us. We're an enormous family.'

Jo and Clare smiled.

I said, 'I have to take my hat off to her really, because to maintain that to your death takes some willpower.'

Retrospectively, however, I think I was wrong about that. I don't think, now, that Catherine's denial of us took some doing. I think it probable that she and Stevie lived so separately from one another that we, Catherine's family, had become genuinely irrelevant, or at the very least simply marginal. Perhaps we were already dead or absent to her, or rather, to Stevie. Perhaps for Stevie even Catherine did not exist.

In all this, there seemed to be a curious symmetry, for inevitably the way we had become for Catherine echoed the way she had become for us. Latterly, there were very few photographs of her in my parents' house because after she turned twenty we had almost no new ones. Even when she was alive, she was a figure more historical than contemporary. There were pictures of the rest of us: weddings, children, parties, dogs, walks, holidays. My mother has one above the fireplace in her bedroom, of Catherine as a baby playing on the lawn. There is also a group picture on my parents' bedroom wall, taken of the family before I was born, formally posed outside the house. But that was it as far as display was concerned. Her childhood and adolescence remained tucked away in photograph albums.

We didn't talk about her much, either. It was too bleak. What is there to say about an absentee family member who wants almost nothing except money, and then only very occasionally, and on her terms only? 'Has anyone heard from Catherine at all this year?' She had removed herself and we had reluctantly taken her lead. What alternative was there? To corner her, harrass her into sharing her life? No. Where there is love and respect that kind of behaviour is categorically not an option.

So she absented herself in her dying, just as she had in her life, and I began to understand that her decision to do so was not about us. Now, it seems patently obvious but at the time it wasn't so. Grief can make one self-absorbed and, if a situation in any way nourishes self-doubt, a little paranoid, too. If the denial of your existence is part of a family member's dying, it's hardly surprising. But I don't think Catherine was trying to hurt us. She wasn't even leaving us. She'd done that years earlier. She was simply dying and I'm certain that any decisions she made at the time were about her and no one else.

Paradoxically, that was both harder and easier to accept than the idea that while she was dying we were unwanted or unnecessary. It was harder because feeling nullified is arguably worse than feeling rejected. It was easier because, frankly, we were used to her solitary nature. So the possibility that we no longer even figured suggests a resolution and stability in Catherine that we had always wished for her but had been afraid she did not possess.

'Was Catherine lonely?' I asked Jo. 'Did she want us to be with her?'

'No,' said Jo. 'She didn't. She didn't want anybody.'

Good. The thought that she might have wanted us and didn't feel she could say so had been haunting me.

'And at Christmas,' said Jo, 'we gave her a present. We give all the patients a present. And she had a Christmas dinner. So you mustn't think she didn't have a Christmas.'

I didn't know what to say.

'I was with Stevie when he died,' said Jo. 'He was in a coma, he'd been unconscious for a couple of days. He was very, very peaceful, just asleep, you know? But I went on talking. He could still hear, so I went on talking to him. And on the day he died, Stevie had had some mouth problems so I went out to get something to tidy up his mouth. When

I came back into the room I realised he wasn't breathing and had died, so I sat down and just spent ten minutes quietly with him.'

I looked at Jo and I felt glad. She had provided for Catherine what I believe she truly wanted as her life closed in: care without fuss. If we'd been with Catherine we would have wished to provide solace and probably to seek it, too, in her physical presence after all those years. I suspect that absolution from the guilt we did not need to feel but could not help might have been on the agenda, too. In retrospect, I'm pleased for all our sakes that Catherine spared us the opportunity to indulge even a little in something ultimately so futile.

I said, 'Thank you. It's good that Stevie was here, that you respected Stevie.'

And Jo and Clare waited patiently while I wept.

Catherine never felt comfortable as a little girl, she cried when she was put into dresses. My mother told me that the last time she bought a dress for Catherine, apart from school uniform, was for our neighbour Candida's wedding. Our other sister was a bridesmaid and in the wedding pictures she looks so pretty, with blonde wispy hair, white organza dress, silk ballet shoes. There's a very beautiful photograph of Candida and her new husband standing at the top of a flight of steps in the garden of the house where they were married, with all the bridesmaids and pageboys spaced out down the steps. Our sister is at the bottom, looking quite angelic. It was she who cried when she was put into trousers.

Whereas Catherine, she almost always looked as uncomfortable in her skin, never mind her clothes, as she probably felt. Even in baby photographs she looks distant, as if at odds with something, and by no means sweetly feminine despite a halo of fluffy gold hair. On the whole, we're a family of pretty good-looking women but Catherine was never beautiful. She looked masculine, always tomboyish. I remember as a child being intrigued and a little put off by her hands for they were so unlike the hands of the other girls and women in the family. There was something inexplicably but incontrovertibly masculine about them.

So for Catherine to become Stevie I thought was a positive evolution. That is not to romanticise her metamorphosis, for it will undoubtedly have had as its source some considerable pain. It would be pretty foolish to believe that to be Stevie while remaining Catherine, biologically, would have been easy or comfortable. But I was so proud of her then, as I sat in that ante-room. My sister: good for her. I was proud of the nurses too, for looking after her psychologically and emotionally in the way that they did: for not mocking or judging her; for being kind to Stevie and not questioning him; above all, for understanding that the maintenance of others' dignity often amounts to no more than the tact and insight to leave them alone.

Jo asked me if I wanted to see the room that Stevie had been in. She explained that he'd wanted to be in a private room, not on a ward.

'It was very important to him to be on his own,' said Jo.

Catherine didn't mix particularly with other patients. I didn't think that especially indicative of a peculiarly isolated personality. How many people are ready to strike up new relationships as they count down the days and hours? When we reached her room somebody else was being settled in so we walked past, but through the square window in the door I was struck by a glancing impression of size and openness.

'Never mind,' said Jo. 'He spent all the time he could in the smoke room. I'll take you there.'

I thought about how and where I had begun my day. It struck me that at seven o'clock that morning I would have been unable not just to anticipate but to imagine the ways in which my perceptions would have to change in the ensuing hours. Catherine, whose frozen hands I had held for the first time in eleven years, was downstairs, awaiting disposal. Stevie, whom I had never met, had smoked his last up here. It was all a little bit much.

The fact that Catherine almost certainly died because she smoked so heavily was not lost on me. There has been no other incidence of breast cancer in our family and though the disease strikes at random, the fact that Catherine chain-smoked from her teens onwards is likely to have been a significant causal factor. Doubtless one could work out approximately what the cost of her hospital care was to the taxpayer, not to mention the cost of her long-term community and psychiatric care. She will have been expensive to maintain, my sister, during her life and during its close. Still, at least nobody at the Bristol Royal Infirmary was trying to persuade terminal cancer patients to adopt pointlessly healthy lifestyles. Apart from instituting some condescending management policy, why would they try? What's the point of forcing people to renounce life-threatening habits if they're days away from death anyway? I've always been a passionate non-smoker but I was never more pleased to see a designated smoking room.

Jo opened the door part-way. The room was no more than a small galley. There was a hospital-issue armchair at one end of it and a picture of a sunflower on the wall above the chair.

'Stevie used to sit in that chair and smoke his roll-ups.'

Catherine chain-smoked roll-ups. In my memories, she is never without one, her restlessness evident in what seemed like a permanent rolling and twisting of tobacco and wafer-thin Rizla papers in her long, bony fingers.

Jo opened the smoke room door further.

Lying on the floor with his head near the door was a young man with very long hair. He was wearing a skirt. He looked, I thought, barely conscious.

'Are you all right, Malcolm?' asked Jo. 'Are you all right there?'

So this was where my sister, known as Stevie, with her crew-cut hair and men's clothes, used to sit and smoke her roll-ups. And now, here was Malcolm, dressed as a woman and with flowing locks, doing exactly the same thing, only prone. There was a clump of long hair on the floor next to the chair where Catherine used to sit. Chemotherapy. It lent the scene some extra pathos that it really could have done without.

Malcolm lifted one thin, pale hand in greeting.

'I'm all right,' he whispered, hoarsely. 'Yeah, I'm fine.'

'All right, then,' said Jo.

Shutting the door, she patted my arm.

'Sorry about that.'

'That's all right.'

'Malcolm likes to smoke. It's a bit of a sight.'

'No, honestly, it's fine.'

A young female patient approached Jo. She was wheeling her portable morphine drip on a trolley.

'There's someone on the floor in the smoke room,' she said.

'Yeah, that's Malcolm. He likes to smoke lying down.'

'Oh, I see.'

'He's all right,' Jo reassured her. 'Honestly. Don't worry about him.'

'Oh, okay then. If he's all right, then I'll go in there.'

She began a slow progress to the smoke room to join Malcolm whom Jo, who had evidently nursed my sister so sensitively, had simply left alone to be the way he wished to be. Maybe Malcolm liked to smoke lying down because it was relaxing. Maybe he was lying down because he felt sick or weak. Whatever the reason, Jo didn't try to budge him or harry him or put him to bed, or jolly him into sitting on a chair. This woman, I thought, is wise and good.

It occurred to me then that if the tabloid newspapers, those great arbiters of bad taste, had seen what I'd just seen, they would have had a field day. The sub-headings are not difficult to imagine: '*Which country do you think the photographs (above) were taken in? India? Romania? China? No, England. Welcome to the Third World NHS. A dying man dressed as a woman lies on the floor of a cancer ward, smoking. You, the UK taxpayer, fund this while the nurses look on.*'

There are many instances in life when nothing is the right thing to do. In such instances, if nothing is the right thing to do, then nothing is a positive action. If those walls of the Bristol Royal Infirmary were the last you would see, the people within them the last among whom you would spend your remaining time, and any decisions you made there the last you would make, would you not wish for the freedom and respect to do so without interference? Would you not wish to be left alone to live as you always had, with your preferences and personal style intact? After all, if you cannot die in peace and whole in hospital, what hope for us all?

Before I left, I had one more question for Jo.

'Did she suffer?'

Jo shook her head.

'No,' she said, 'the pain control was good. She had a little diamorphine drip, and a button that she could press herself, to up the dose when she needed it.'

I sighed and leaned against the corridor wall. That wasn't quite the answer I was after. I felt suddenly enervated, shivery and a little shaky.

I said, 'Apart from the pain, how was she otherwise? It

sounds like a stupid question but was she – ' I stalled, 'was she all right?' I couldn't find the words to describe what I meant. 'Was she really all right?'

But Jo understood.

'Yes,' she said, and she touched my arm lightly with her hand. 'She was. She was really all right.'

Location, Location

I'd agreed to meet my husband and daughter in a coffee bar around the corner from Maudlin Street and the mortuary. Clare was in a high chair playing with a biscotti wrapped in cellophane. Andrew had already eaten and moved on to the newspapers. He was sweet and kind when I arrived. I could tell that he was expecting me to cry because he had that look that husbands get when they think their wives will cry; a mixture of concern and slight panic. He was probably surprised that I didn't.

But in truth, I was beginning to feel numb. I ordered a tuna and pasta salad and some olive bread. It's not my favourite kind of food at the best of times but it was hours since breakfast and I usually eat like a horse. I couldn't eat anything. I felt sick and wondered for a minute or two whether I might be. I tried a bit of food but there was no flavour and too much texture. My mouth was ash-dry. While I might have felt fully alive after my visit to the mortuary, the oncology ward and smoke room had reduced my appetite for blankly cheerful coffee bar fare.

We set off for Catherine's flat and of course got lost on the way. We found ourselves snarled up in the one-way system and baffled by the many re-developments that weren't on our outdated Bristol map. My mother had thoughtfully provided us with a photocopy of the relevant page from her more recent map but the quality of the copy was poor and it was impossible to read. So we stopped at a garage and were sent back the way we'd come. We wound down the window and asked strangers for directions and they sucked air through their teeth and said things like:

'First right, second left, there's a dog-leg bend, go round it and then straight across the roundabout, mind the traffic bumps, take the – let me see, one, two, three – third, no, fourth set of traffic lights, there's a pub on the corner, DON'T go left there, wait until you see a petrol station on your left with a sharp left turn straight after it, well, you don't want that turning . . .'

And in the end, as people do, we got there, somehow.

Though it was only lunchtime the light was already fading.

The block of flats that Catherine lived in was brick, three-storey, built in the 1930s. Catherine lived at number 38. The only time I ever visited her in Bristol, when I was twenty-one, she was living at number 15, and then all the walkways around the flats were outdoors and the building was exceptionally bleak and forbidding. It had changed in the years since. It was done up in the eighties or early nineties, by the look of it. All the walkways had been enclosed so that the external corridors were now inside. Doors and windows had been replaced. The roof was in good nick. The clouds above it were dark with moisture and I remembered something my mother had said about bringing a torch. The electricity in the flat had long since been cut off.

I got out of the car and rang the bell of the caretaker's flat, which was on the ground floor. The caretaker, Steve Shepherd, appeared, quite a well-built man in his forties, very friendly and jangling a large bunch of keys. We greeted one another and he unlocked the main door to the part of the block where Catherine had lived. A metal sign on the wall announced, Flats 36–57. The staircase was dark grey and very clean. The banisters were grey, brushed steel, their effect modern and suburban. There was new brick in the stairwell and circular windows allowing in a lot of light. If the stairs had led instead to a set of small-town solicitors' or architects' offices I wouldn't have been surprised.

Up one short flight of steps and Steve began jangling his keys again. With the precision of a blind man he selected one from the many in his hand and lifted it to the door before us. Suddenly there it was, flat number 38, and I wasn't mentally prepared for it, was immediately feverish with fear. This experience was the antithesis of going to see Catherine's body. Then, I had nice Mr Carpenter to pace me through everything. Now, the timing felt all wrong. There was her door, a dull, dark-grey painted door suggesting little, revealing nothing.

There are few things so symbolic as a door, and a door to the home of a long-lost relation has its own peculiar resonance. For years I imagined myself knocking on it, and for years resisted the urge to travel to Bristol to do just that. Sometimes I fantasised about the door being opened and Catherine smiling and inviting me in. I dreamed that just one visit from me might subtly alter the world beyond the door, tip the balance towards a desire for more contact, a wish for regular visits with tea and cake. At other times, I imagined the door closing behind me and Catherine refusing to let me leave, Catherine violent. In fact, when I was in my twenties my mother had made me promise her that I would not visit Catherine alone, so afraid was she of what might happen if I did. After years of seeing this very door in my imagination alone the shock was profound. Much greater than the fear of seeing Catherine dead was the prospect of seeing where she had lived.

Momentarily, Steve faltered.

'We didn't realise the flat was so . . .' he trailed off.

I said, 'Don't worry.'

But he was embarrassed all the same.

'I'll be downstairs,' he said. 'Just come and knock on my door when you've finished.'

And then he left me there.

Well, of course he did. What did I expect?

I made it half way into the entrance hall, which was fairly big and empty. Some jackets in various shades of beige and grey hung on hooks on the wall. They looked stiff and lifeless, as if they'd been there for an exceedingly long time. They were thin, lacking warmth or comfort. On the wall beside the jackets was a white box with a red panic button and a long cord with a red triangular handle; a recent addition, I guessed. By the front door was a poster of a smudgy rainbow with the words, *Do you really know who you are?* splashed across it in white paint.

There was a noise. I'm not sure what it was, probably the water system or something, but it frightened me. It was a low, constant hum, almost a buzz. And it wasn't just the noise, there was something else, too. It was a presence, the most forbidding presence I have felt anywhere, ever. Of what or whom it was I do not know.

I took a few steps further into the hall, from where I could see in to Catherine's main room.

In the far, diagonal corner of the room was a mattress on the floor with a sleeping-bag and an assortment of covers on top of it. Still curled as they'd been left, when she quit her bed some weeks earlier, the shape of a human body hunched in sleep, cold or pain was apparent.

I could go no further. I was terrified.

*　　*　　*

My mother had visited Catherine's flat a few days earlier. She had tried to discourage me from going there myself.

'Why?' I asked her.

There was a longish silence before she spoke again.

She said, 'It's distressing.'

'So? That's not a reason not to go.'

'I don't want you to be upset any more than you need to be.'

'I'd be more upset if I didn't go. I want to see where she lived.'

My mother sighed.

'That's fair enough,' she concurred, adding, 'I feel that all of Catherine's problems were contained in that flat. It reminded me of Dorian Gray.'

Dorian Gray is a fictional creation of Oscar Wilde's, who lives a free and somewhat dissipated life, all the while remaining young and lovely. He never ages. However, he keeps a portrait of himself locked away in the attic of his house and the picture grows old and disfigured, reflecting his true physical and moral demise.

'What do you mean it reminded you of Dorian Gray?' I asked.

'Well, I think the flat reflected a lot of Catherine that wouldn't have been obviously visible, or at least as marked, in her exterior life. And I think she'd deteriorated. Her previous flat, compared with this one, was positively pristine. There is not one surface, and I mean not one, on which you could put Clare.'

I had thought she was exaggerating. I'd packed a rug in the car for Clare to roll around on while we sorted Catherine's stuff.

In awe of the dying light and the steady hum from somewhere I knew not, I backed out of the hall, turned, and bolted into the stairwell. I called out to Andrew, rather desperately.

'Darling, can you come up? I need you here, I can't go in on my own.'

But he was already on his way up the stairs, with Clare in her pram. Mercifully, she was still asleep.

When he reached the flat he parked the pram in the hallway and walked without hesitation into the main room.

I loved him very deeply for that, loved him for being so much a man, so straightforward and unafraid.

'Wow,' he exhaled.

I cowered in the hallway next to Clare and her pram.

'Wow,' he said again.

My mother was right. I had focused upon Catherine's bed, zoomed in on it like a telephoto lens. But it was the bed's surroundings that had sent me backwards out of the flat. I remembered my mother's words: 'There is not one surface on which you could put Clare.' There was not one surface, full stop. There was no furniture, not a chair, not a table, nothing. And yet the room was not empty. The room was almost as far from being empty as it is possible to be. It was so full that you couldn't see the floor at all. You couldn't even guess where best to tread in the hope of finding solid ground beneath.

I surveyed the area immediately in front of me and absorbed what was visible, the jagged top layer of a derangement so profound that I doubt I will ever see its like again. I looked at the things I would have to walk over in order simply to enter the room, looked at what I might clear if I took only two strides.

Broken biscuits, crusts of bread and desiccated cheese lying in amongst papers, old shoes, empty bottles of washing-up liquid, paints, felt tips. A copy of *Soldier* magazine floating on some non-matching plimsolls. An army-style canvas shoulder bag, thick with grease. Lots of fake pot plants, maybe twenty of them, mostly white; some were propped against other things, others jettisoned into the mix at all angles. Piles and piles of Catherine's own paintings of Tibetan monks and the Dalai Lama. Small patterned rugs, tossed, curled up, concealing other things. A red-lettered No Smoking sign. A Police Constabulary shield attached to a wall plaque, an empty picture frame in imitation gold-leaf, a pink pig alarm clock, a Rubik's cube, a brass lampshade shaped like a partially opened umbrella, upside down in the turmoil like an upturned parasol on a storm-blasted beach. A brass crucifix on a plinth, a brass ornament of the Taj Mahal, a white china Madonna, customised with a strand of small, turquoise rosary beads. An ornamental football cup decorated with the words Bristol City in red. A silver bell with green foliage around the top, clearly a Christmas decoration. A bottle of prescription pills, a hurricane lamp, empty packets of Kodak 35mm film.

And beneath it all was more of the same. Lifting the corners of rugs and pictures I de-stabilised more lamps and shoes, tipped over pens and papers, discovered more tins, boxes, flowers, clocks. Another layer, concealing another layer, concealing another.

I took those two strides and beneath my feet things crunched, subsided or creaked. I was aiming for the far corner of the room, where Catherine's bed was. I could see now that there were two mattresses, one on top of another, the lower one patterned with blue flowers, now greying, the upper one striped blue and white. On top of them was the blue nylon sleeping-bag I had noticed earlier, and a thin gold eiderdown with bits of flock coming out at the seams. On top of the eiderdown was an assortment of blankets and a purple patterned sheet. Where normally a pillow would have been there were cushions: one was dark green,

one deep pink and two gold, all grimy. A brown teddy bear
with a white nose lay near the wall, green and white rosary
beads around its neck. It was carefully tucked under a blue
cotton baby blanket. It had been put to bed, lovingly by
the look of it. There was a man's black beanie-style hat at
its feet. A grubby white fluffy toy dog lay haphazardly to
one side of the hat.

Beside the bed was an alarm clock, two empty packets of
Mini Cheddars and an empty carton of semi-skimmed milk.
There were containers and packets of Nurofen, Pot Noodles,
Brasso, cheese, prescription medicines and joss sticks, all of
them now empty. A collection of cassette tapes was in a red
metal biscuit tin. I put the tin on the end of the bed to take
away with me and picked up a handful of tapes to look at:
Verdi, *La Traviata*; Louis Jordan, *How 'Bout That*; *Elvis
Presley Live*; *The Essential Pavarotti*. Fake roses, in pale and
deep pinks, were littered between nightlights and opened,
discarded books. I turned over the books: John Wesley's *The
Message Today*; one entitled *Muscular Dystrophy*; another,
Man Eaters of Kumaon and The Temple Tiger. There were
other books, too, books about dogs, the military, and once-
glossy hardbacks that might in other households have been
referred to as 'coffee-table' books. Beneath them were
scrunched-up papers: a letter from the WSPA, thanking
Catherine for a donation to a campaign to stop bear-baiting
in Turkey; another, similar, letter from Guide Dogs For The
Blind.

Catherine had fashioned a couple of bedside tables, one
from a suitcase covered with a brass tray, the other from an
old trunk. On the brass tray was a lamp with a frilly, gold
lampshade and a further collection of tapes, loose this time.
Next to the tray was another gold lampshade on its side and
more packets of pills, some empty, some unopened. It was
odd that in amongst all this chaos the drugs could manage

to look deliberately discarded but they did. There was something about their disposition that suggested they had been cast aside intentionally, in frustration or even anger. Side by side, facing the bed, a small Buddha and tiny plastic panda sat amongst some abandoned steroid tablets.

On the trunk was a radio-cassette player and more cassette tapes, a china cart-horse and photographs cut out from newspapers, of people mostly, ordinary people. Next to the trunk was a white china sphinx and yet more gold lamps and lampshades. There were more of her pictures, this time of motorcyclists and Tibetan warriors. Lots of old newspapers, mainly *The Times*. A white moped crash helmet, with a Bristol City sticker on it. More radios and clocks. A heater stood against the wall but was clearly out of commission. Covered in thick dust, it was largely obscured by objects and stacks of pictures.

Catherine's badge collection was here, too, on a large piece of chipboard. I remembered the collection from my last ever visit to her. She had been very proud of it. The badges were pinned to the chipboard in approximate rows. I glanced at the top row:

Cat Lovers Against the Bomb; British Meat's Got The Lot; Join the Rejects and Get Yourself Killed; Bristol City Museum and Art Gallery; All This and Brains Too; The Boomtown Rats; The Wildfowl Trust; I am 23; Only An Idiot Would Wear This Badge; Happy Winter; Alfa Romeo. One had a limerick-style ditty in tiny print: *There was a young man from Kent, Who swallowed a set of encyclopaedias. His mother said, 'Ken, what have you done – They were for supper!'*

I pulled my camera from my jacket pocket and took a couple of photographs, wondering all the while whether they'd come out. I am neither religious nor especially superstitious about the supernatural and yet I felt fairly certain that Catherine would find a way to interfere with them: either her spirit would screw up the film processing or, when they were eventually developed, she would feature in the photographs themselves. It wouldn't have surprised me in the least bit if in one of them she were to appear, sitting on the floor or on her bed, meditating, palms upturned, supple and cross-legged as I remembered her. I dreaded her phantom appearance. I longed for it, too.

Perhaps it was there all along in her home, which my husband and I now picked our way across in shock and awe. Certainly, I had never before had such an overwhelming sense of an absent person. The magnitude of it was breathtaking. I was distinctly aware of pain, menace, fury, sadness and despair. I didn't feel anything positive. No humour, no light. The flat was dark. There was deep dust everywhere. The room smelt of decay.

Already desperate for some respite I crunched over my dead sister's things and went to stand in the stairwell, away from the intense gloom of the flat's interior. I looked down the stairs to the main entrance and there I noticed a woman getting out of a car parked next to ours.

I knew who she was. Jo Fleming, Catherine's GP. She and my parents had been in touch with each other since Catherine's death, and I had then contacted her, too, to ask if she might consider meeting me when I was in Bristol. She had known Catherine for eighteen years. She would surely have light to shed upon this appalling darkness. I had been very nervous of asking, though, and had fully expected her to say no. Instead, she had agreed readily. Then there was the question of where we should meet. The circumstances didn't exactly lend themselves to an obvious location. Why not at the flat, she had suggested, as you'll be there. Then, I had no way of knowing that there were a million good reasons why not.

Jo had dark shoulder-length hair. In her forties, pretty and neat but in no way ostentatious, she looked both unthreatening and imperturbable. She seemed very familiar with where she was. There was something automatic about the way in which she got out of her car and approached the building that made me think she'd been to it many times before. Had she been a lot or come only latterly, when Catherine was very ill? Perhaps she had other patients in the building. I wondered how she felt about coming to meet me there.

Not altogether sure, I decided, as she climbed the stairs and took my outstretched hand, when she reached the top.

'Hello,' she said calmly, but she didn't quite meet my gaze. I couldn't tell if she was embarrassed, reluctant or shy.

'Hello,' I replied. 'Thank you for coming. It's kind of you.'

She shrugged. I think she just felt awkward.

I gestured to her to enter the flat ahead of me. Her shoulders were slightly hunched in her jacket, betraying either the reserve I thought I had already detected or a reaction to the cold. Otherwise, I could read nothing in her demeanour.

'This is my husband, Andrew,' I said, as the two of them shook hands. 'Andrew, this is Jo Fleming. And this,' I indicated the pram, 'is Clare.'

Jo smiled politely in Clare's direction.

Andrew and I had already discussed Jo and I'd decided I wanted to see her alone.

'Right,' he said. 'I think I'm going to get some air, leave you two to have a chat. How long will you need, do you think?'

I looked at Jo for guidance but she offered none. She looked at the floor.

I said, 'Oh, twenty-five minutes, half an hour, I'm sure that's enough.'

'Well, I'll go for a walk, then.'

'There's a department store nearby,' Jo ventured, 'a DIY store that's got a café.'

'Good,' said Andrew. 'That'll do fine.'

'Sounds like the perfect combination for you,' I said. 'You can handle lots of different tools and drink coffee.'

'I will,' he said, and he kissed me goodbye.

I listened to the sound of him bumping Clare down the stairs in her pram.

Jo and I stood in the centre of Catherine's room and were silent.

I felt immensely awkward. Here was the person with whom Catherine was most familiar, as far as we knew, the person she talked to and trusted. This was the person who was as close to being everything to Catherine that we hadn't been but would have liked to be. Though I felt very grateful to her for coming I was angry, too. I was angry that it was her and not us. I felt envious of her relationship with Catherine. I felt inadequate.

I was also frightened of being judged by her. I had no idea what Catherine had or hadn't said to Jo about her life or her family. And whatever Catherine had said, Jo wouldn't necessarily have had any way of knowing what was true. I wondered what Jo had been told, what she knew, what she guessed and what she believed. Much of what Catherine maintained, like being followed by the Secret Services, was clearly implausible. However, one of the problems for the mentally ill is that very often their version of events is regarded as questionable simply because they are ill. Sometimes they are telling the truth, however unlikely. So if you believed, as Catherine did, that you'd been tortured and raped in a foreign prison, then whether or not you had been would be somewhat irrelevant when taking into account the effect of that belief upon your personality. If the maintenance of a conviction impinges upon your life and behaviour, to an extent its truth lies in its consequences, not its origins.

Many things that were real for Catherine could be neither tested nor proved. She may or may not have been tortured and raped but she believed that she had been and she displayed many of the signs of distress common to tortured people, although some of those signs are common to schizophrenics, too. In that sense she was a tortured person, whether or not the original sins had happened in a prison or in her mind only. The fact that her reality was a complicated blend of fact and fantasy did not differentiate her from the rest of us. What set her apart was the degree of distortion involved in the mix.

Still, it felt like Judgement Day there amongst the toys and broken clocks and discarded shoes. There I stood in what I had hoped when dressing that morning was as neutral an ensemble as possible: neat black trousers, flat black ankle boots, a warm jersey and a mountaineering jacket. In these particular and peculiar circumstances, I didn't want to look too girlish or too prosperous. I wanted to look feminine, sensible and sympathetic. I wanted categorically not to look like the sort of woman you'd want instinctively to tell to get lost, just for being in better physical and financial health than her late sister. In the middle of that terrifying chaos I could not stop worrying, What is this woman, Jo, thinking about my family? Does she despise us?

Perhaps I should have asked her but I lacked the courage, and anyway it wasn't appropriate. There were so many other questions I knew I wanted to ask and I had no idea where to start.

I said as much.

'You should have written them down,' Jo said calmly, with a faint smile.

'I know I should have done. I didn't.'

I asked her about Catherine's desire to die without letting

us know. There wasn't much to say. Catherine wanted to die alone.

'She had her own life,' said Jo. 'She had her life here in Bristol.'

For a moment I was deeply comforted. Catherine had her own life and it included other things. It was full. Every life is necessarily full, of something. There is no such thing as an empty life, it's an impossibility.

Jo said, 'Your father's a GP, isn't he.'

'He was. He does research now and he's an artist, too, he always has been.'

'Catherine talked a bit about your parents and about the family. She was very devoted to you. She spoke a lot about you.'

I was taken aback. What could she have found to talk about except a very old past? Surely not the me of my letters, those hopeless letters I had written to her; letters of the kind, I realise now, that you might politely write to a great-aunt. I very much doubt she had anything to say about my books either. I sent them to her and she acknowledged the first of them with warm congratulations but I don't imagine she actually read them. I suppose she might have done. She might even have read *Man Eaters of Kumaon* and *The Temple Tiger* for that matter. Anything is possible.

'I think it was easy for her to love me,' I said, 'because I was no threat. I wasn't involved in her life in the way the others were. I wasn't close to her in the way they were. They knew her much better and for longer and I wasn't part of that. I was a later, fifth child and there was quite a gap between me and the next one up. Anyway, it was probably easier for me to have a straightforward relationship with her because I was little and she was simply an adored older sister.'

'Well, you were an idolised younger sister.'

Had Catherine idolised me? Maybe she had. She certainly never knew me as an adult or even very much as an adolescent. The last time I saw her was for a couple of hours or so when I was twenty-one. The time before that I was fifteen and she came home for a few nights. That's a fairly reasonable basis for an unrealistic long-distance relationship.

I don't think I idolised her but I've had to think about it. It's true that it is much easier to be understanding of a sometimes unpredictable, difficult and frightening individual once they're not actually there. A bereaved person may well be more disposed to sympathy for a dead relation than someone still facing ongoing demands that they don't know how to meet.

I knew, however, that I was not standing in that cold, dark flat with a woman I did not know in order to hero-worship my sister now that she was dead. I was simply in search of her, so elusive had she been when she was alive. I could not let her go without an effort. I did not want to claim her, only to locate her. I wanted to know who and where she had been. Her frozen feet, the smoke room, the broken objects amongst which she lived, I wanted to take them on and find out what they meant and where they belonged in my own life, if they belonged at all. I wanted to find in them the family member we had lost and preserve something of her essence for good. I wanted something to hold on to. She was part of me, even if it was a progressively small part. I could not let her disappear like a stone into deep water.

I said, 'I gather she'd been living as Stevie for a while.'

'For many years.'

'Do you know how many?'

'Oh gosh,' said Jo, 'I'm not sure. About eight, I think. She found her periods very disturbing and I'd given her something to stop them some years ago. She found being reminded that she was a woman very distressing. She didn't feel like a woman and she didn't want them, and I think . . .'

Jo paused for a minute and then she said, 'I think that was the right thing to do.'

I said, 'I'm sure it was.'

Jo wanted reassurance, or at least I thought she did and that was enough for me. I was no longer the only person in the room seeking something. I had something to offer, too. The conversation finally opened up a little, like a stiff gate giving way just enough to allow you to squeeze beyond it.

'Catherine was very distressed by having breast cancer,' said Jo. 'I think it's one of the reasons she didn't present with it until it was really too late. She had a lump for over a year before telling me.'

'Why didn't she tell you?'

'I think she thought she would be mocked.'

'For having a cancer in the breast?'

'Yes.'

'What, like it was too female for her?'

'Yes. She was also afraid of getting ill and afraid of the treatment, of the pain.'

'Was she afraid of dying?'

'Yes, she was. She didn't want to die. She was enjoying her life.'

Oh, how normal. My poor sister.

The light had faded further and the temperature was dropping. Jo gestured mildly around the room.

She said, 'What's happening to the flat? What's happening to Cathy's things?'

'It's being cleared, I think. My parents are in charge of that.'

I didn't want to admit to her what I knew, that my parents were finished here, that the Council was coming to clear the rest of the things.

I said, 'My mother's already been and taken quite a lot. I've come to take some things, too, I think, but I'm not sure. I'm not sure what to take.'

Jo's poise seemed momentarily to waver.

'Well,' she said, with some firmness, 'there are a lot of things here that were very special to Cathy.'

I felt a flash of anger but much more gratitude. Here was something concrete. All these objects and perhaps some means of classifying them.

'What are they? Will you tell me? Because I don't know.' I was almost pleading.

Jo said, looking around the room, 'Well, polar bears were important.'

There were a lot of polar bears. From where I was standing I could see two soft ones and several china ones.

My mother had already taken quite a few of Catherine's soft animals. They were mostly teddy bears but there was also a badger and a donkey. 'Something to hold on to, something to be comforted by,' is what she had said about them. Possibly that's the function they served. But who's to say that Catherine didn't simply like them? I didn't know.

Anyway, polar bears were special.

Jo turned and picked up a red and white football scarf from the floor. She said, 'Football was important. Cathy used to wear this a lot.'

I took it from her, I almost snatched it.

'Fine. That's fine, I'll take it.'

I put it in the heavy-duty Waitrose bag I'd brought, one of several in which to put things. *Bag For Life*, it stated on the side. 'Whose life?' my mother once asked, drily, when I pilfered some of hers to go shopping with.

Jo continued.

'Badges were important. She collected badges.'

'I knew that. I knew that already.'

I thought back to my visit to Catherine, when she was living in her previous flat. I was twenty-one, Catherine was thirty-four. It was the last time I saw her alive. She showed the badges to my mother and me then, and I remembered not knowing what to say. I was embarrassed by her child-like pride in the collection, upset that her life was reduced to this. I was polite. I showed an interest. But I suppose I failed to mask my shock and awkwardness and I think she must have sensed them. I think they must have been what she was alluding to when she wrote to my mother after-wards asking her not to bring me to see her again. *It's too painful*, she wrote. My mother thought that was because Catherine could see in me all the things she would never be. I don't. I think she saw in me someone who no longer accepted her for who she was. Time had removed her spon-taneous baby sister and replaced her with a guarded young woman. Time had betrayed Catherine, like so much else.

Catherine was in a Michael Jackson phase then, I remember. I can recall as if it were an hour ago the news-paper pictures and posters of the singer stuck firmly to her sitting-room wall, with no space between them. It is the most powerful visual memory I have of her in her own surround-ings. Actually, it is the only one I have: in all the others, she is at the family home or on a family holiday, or in hospital. There were probably well over a hundred of those Michael Jackson pictures in that flat, interspersed with National Geographic-style photographs of wolves and bears, and CND stickers. No teenager could have come close to making that wall look both more and less like a teenager's wall.

I sat next to my mother on Catherine's bed, which doubled up as a sofa, staring at the wall in some disbelief. The bed itself was beautifully made, with a checked wool rug on top and a lot of soft toys at its head. The kitchen off the main room was narrow, bleak and dark. The naked light bulb that hung from the ceiling was inoperative. There was nothing at all in the kitchen to lift the spirits and certainly nothing of substance to eat but Catherine still produced mugs of tea and a plate of biscuits. She laughed a lot, for no reason I could discern, and muttered to herself and chain-smoked. But compared with what I was standing in now, again my mother was right: that flat had been positively pristine and more to the point, Catherine had been functioning reasonably well within it.

Jo looked around further. She was on a roll now.

'This bag was important,' she announced, dangling a rectangular leather satchel from her hand, 'and there was another one, a canvas one, and a brown leather jacket.'

'A brown jacket, right. I'll look for it.'

'And the paintings. Paintings are important.'

'I know that.'

Jo picked up a second football scarf. It was similar to the first.

'Everything's important, really.'

'Yes.'

I began to wonder how much more I could stand of all this. I took the leather satchel and began gathering the polar bears. I took the two soft ones from her bed, one pretty new, one elderly. Both were grey with dirt, or love.

I removed the china ones from an upturned box covered in material next to her bed. It was clearly a small shrine of some sort. Apart from some Tibetan-style holy objects, the box also supported her tape-recorder and a tin in which there were some remains of Digestive biscuits. I looked at them and thought, I hate Digestive biscuits. I considered the tin, decided to leave it, and scooped up another football scarf. Surely I won't take all these scarves home, I thought; I'll have to decide which ones to leave.

I turned back to Jo.

'Was she unhappy?' I asked her. 'Was she unhappy in herself? That really troubles me. I mean, I hate the thought but please be honest with me. I can take it.'

I could, too, though I had a feeling that too many questions like that were not necessarily a good idea, at least not today, not in this room. What good could the answers do now? On the other hand, having embarked upon this journey towards my sister there wasn't going to be an obvious point at which to stop and decide to turn back.

Who was I kidding? There wasn't any chance of turning back. Not now.

Jo looked at me directly.

'No, she wasn't unhappy. Obviously, there were times when she was more difficult to deal with than others but she was generally cheerful. She was quite bouncy at times.'

'But this is a sad room.'

Jo looked around.

She said, 'Well, I don't know. I don't know. It's got . . . it's got her paintings. It's a very creative room.'

I fumbled to agree with her.

'Yes. I see that. You're right, it is. You're right.'

I wanted to see it that way although I didn't. I felt I'd made a terrible blunder. I had made a judgement about the flat and therefore about my sister to someone who knew her better than I did. I had imposed my own values on to it and compared it with some imaginary idea of the way in which Catherine lived. Hadn't I?

We talked some more. Jo said that Catherine didn't keep appointments, which was no surprise. She was supposed to have fortnightly injections and she didn't always turn up for them, and if she went a while without them she became less stable. But if Jo, or Maria, the practice nurse, saw Catherine in the street, or in the surgery car park, they'd try to encourage her to come in, and they'd give her the injection there and then. And if Catherine was in the waiting-room they always made sure she came ahead of other patients, that she wasn't kept hanging around.

'Was she aggressive or hostile towards you?' I asked. 'Because she used to be towards us, sometimes.'

'No, she wasn't,' Jo replied, 'although she fell out with Maria a couple of times. But she never fell out with me.'

There was a noise in the hallway, and I called out.

'Andrew?'

Two men put their heads around the door. Neither of them was Andrew. They were both considerably overweight and wearing navy blue overalls. One was shorter than his companion.

'Hello,' I said. 'Can I help you?'

'We've come to clear the flat,' said the shorter man.

I had not the faintest idea what he was talking about.

'I'm sorry?'

'We've come to clear the flat,' he repeated, dully. 'We've got instructions to clear the flat.'

I was perplexed.

I said, 'I understood it wasn't happening for several days, or even weeks.'

'Oh no,' said the man, 'No, we've come to do it today. The tenant's gone, so we've got to come in and clear it.'

'I know the tenant's gone. I'm her sister.'

'Well, where is she?'

He looked around the room casually. Did he think she might be lurking under some old shoes and tins of poster paint?

'She's dead.'

He grunted, shifting a bit of detritus with one foot.

'So when's she coming back, then?' he asked.

'You tell me,' I snapped, incredulous. 'She's dead.'

'Oh,' he said, blankly. 'Well, we've got to clear it.'

There was a pause. Then he turned to Jo.

'Who are you?' he asked.

Jo said, quite crisply, 'I'm the doctor.'

She was protecting me, or Catherine.

He turned back to me, obdurate.

'Well, what do you want me to do?' he demanded. 'What do you want to do?'

I looked at Jo for help. She looked at the floor.

I said, 'This is not a good time. I'm afraid you'll have to go away and come back another time. You'd better go and talk to Steve Shepherd, the caretaker. But you absolutely cannot clear this flat today. Okay?'

'Uh.'

The men shrugged, grumbled and finally departed, just as Andrew re-appeared, with Clare in the pram.

'Who were they?' he asked.

'I'll tell you later.'

'I'd better go,' said Jo.

'Of course,' I said. 'Thank you for coming. I really appreciate it.'

She smiled, warmly this time. Perhaps she had felt as awful as I had.

'Look,' I said, 'I'm sorry if I've been a bit off, I just . . . it's just . . . well, you know.'

'Yes.'

'You're coming to the funeral,' I said, adding, 'Is that right?'

'Yes,' said Jo. 'If I can, I will.'

You won't come, I thought. GPs can't go to funerals all the time otherwise they'd spend half their lives at them. You won't come.

Jo shook hands with Andrew.

'Thank you for coming,' Andrew said. 'I know Mary was really pleased that you could.'

'It's nothing,' said Jo. 'Really.'

And she left the flat as she had entered it, quietly and with her self-possession intact. Any relief she might have felt at the prospect of being outside those four walls once more was not discernible, her composure apparently unruffled by the tempest they contained.

The Writing On the Wall

There was no obvious way to proceed. Any order that may have existed for Catherine would have been impossible for anyone else to detect. It was hopeless trying to move without treading on things and it was difficult to see what it was you were treading on. I knew the process of finding anything I wanted was going to be entirely haphazard, that it would not be a process at all but instead a muddled and muddling endeavour.

I did try. I attempted to be methodical. I picked a few things up, put them into a plastic bag. The scarves, the polar bears; the smaller one had a Winnie the Pooh watch strapped to its paw. I thought I'd try and take a bit of everything: art, music, some animals and clothes, some watches. I gathered up the cassette tapes from beside Catherine's bed and put them together in a box. I put the box in a separate bag. I would listen to her music. One day, I would listen to her music and hear what she had heard, experience what she had chosen. I now knew where she had listened to it herself.

Throughout my search, I was looking beyond what I could see and searching for what I couldn't, for what I wanted most. I wanted letters, cards, evidence of our family. I wanted also some evidence of a life that extended beyond the confines of this terrible, schizophrenic jail. My mother had found almost none and I'd felt sure that if she'd only looked further, she could have done. I understood now I was here how unrealistic that was. I don't even know if it would have been possible to recognise any evidence if we'd come across it. I don't know if it was under my nose the whole time, if a lot of what was in that room was in fact quite normal but rendered insane by its setting.

'Bloody hell,' I sighed.

'I know,' said Andrew.

'I mean, where on earth do I start? What do we take? What do we leave? Nothing in here makes any sense.'

Andrew was bent over, sifting through objects in the centre of the room. He stood up and paused for a minute. One of my husband's many qualities is his ability to think rationally in highly charged situations.

'I don't know,' he said. 'Look, you can see that the room has specific areas. There's her Tibetan shrine. There's nearly all her football stuff, it looks like another shrine, doesn't it, a football shrine. Over there by the door is where most of the paints and pens seem to be.'

I looked vaguely around me. Sure enough, visible in one part of the room was Catherine's collection of poster paints and oils, or at least the part of the collection that I could detect. Some tins of Galt's powder colours nestled between defunct carriage clocks and a couple of hurricane lamps. Amongst a number of plumply-filled plastic carrier bags were some brushes and palette knives. Their organisation was slightly undermined by the presence of another greying teddy bear, which lay across them, carefully wrapped in a red candlewick bedspread.

'I mean, it's not exactly obvious, that's for sure,' Andrew conceded. 'But I think at some point before it got so bad in here she will have had quite a definite sense of what went where, and why.'

I looked over towards the football area. He was right, it did look like a shrine. Despite the fact that it was now mixed up with many other things you could still make out distinct football paraphernalia of all kinds: cups, shields, plaques, scarves, rosettes. Some of the cups and rosettes had evidently been put on display, lined up in rows that once were orderly but had since become irregular. Scarves had been draped around the cups. *City 1 Rovers 0* was written at a diagonal on the wall in Catherine's unmistakable spaced-out lettering.

The dozens of pictures immediately surrounding the football scene were Catherine's own pictures of players. All of them were meaty men built more like Maori prop forwards than provincial English footballers, with short legs, bulging thighs and pectorals, and faces constructed of slabs and planes of interlocking muscle. There was a quality of vague and non-specific violence to the pictures. I couldn't work out why that was, and couldn't decide whether they were supposed to look aggressive or were simply representative of masculinity and strength as Catherine perceived it, or a bit of both. Most of the men were poised to kick a ball suspended in mid-air: a few were dribbling the balls, their heads turned in the direction of other imaginary players to whom they could pass. They had some energy but little individual expression.

'Do you think Jo knew how Catherine was living?' Andrew asked.

'She must have done,' I replied.

'Not necessarily.'

I said, 'She seemed pretty unfazed by it all.'

'She was her doctor.'

'Yes, but that doesn't mean she'd been here a lot. Still, perhaps it was a shock to her, too. Perhaps she just hid her reaction well.'

'It didn't seem to be a shock to her.'

'No,' I agreed. 'It didn't.'

I thought about Jo's remark, 'It's a very creative room,' and I experienced a wild, passionate surge of anger. Either

Jo was right, in which case there must have been something very wrong with me that I couldn't see it that way, couldn't see creativity as the room's main feature. Or she was wrong, in which case, how could she let it go on? How on earth could anyone who knew that Catherine lived like this allow it to continue? How could they allow her to be in this place, festering alone, ill-fed, dying?

I made a vow to try and talk to Jo again. Now, there was so much more that I wanted to ask her. Now, I was filled with particular questions, questions I would never have had before today. Had she been complicit in the manner of Catherine's demise or respectful of her desire for privacy? If she'd left Catherine to it, was that good or bad, right or wrong? I was shaking with fury, shock and confusion. I packed some more bags, unaware of the meaning, if meaning there was, of almost everything I put inside them. I worked silently alongside Andrew for half an hour or so and slowly, slowly I calmed down. Gradually, it occurred to me that Jo had probably only done what we, Catherine's family, had done. She had left her alone. She had followed her lead. She would have been all too aware that you cannot force a patient into hospital or foist Social Services onto an individual who won't open the door to anyone. You cannot make someone take the medicine you prescribe. Jo would have understood that to push someone on the edge would more than likely tip them over it and away from you, and from any support you had to offer.

Perhaps Jo hadn't known as much as I thought about this place. Perhaps she had and had lived with the dilemmas.

It was exhausting, just thinking about it all.

Hanging on the wall at the head of Catherine's bed was a musical instrument of some sort. It was garlanded with a string of Hawaiian-style flowers made of silk. And hanging by the window was a small electronic keyboard and a brass bugle. I noticed a recorder at the foot of the bed. Musical notes had been drawn on the wall: like everything else that Catherine had drawn upon the walls, they were denoted in thick, black marker pen.

Across the room was football. Here, right next to her bed just like the tape collection, was music. Music had been so much a part of Catherine's life. The Beatles, Bob Dylan, The Rolling Stones. Mozart, Beethoven, Bach, Handel. She loved Bluegrass music, folk and jazz. And then, later, there were all those Indian chants and Tibetan prayers. Each of us in the family had had music lessons. Between us we played the piano, flute, trombone and violin. But Catherine had surpassed us all by taking her skills one step further and transferring her allegiance from the piano to a full-sized church organ, an overwhelming instrument requiring simultaneous use of hands and feet. It required mastery not just of the keyboard – two keyboards – but of pedals and stops, too. To me, the piano is a well-tempered creature, the organ a terrifying, gargantuan beast. When taken as a child into vast French cathedrals, I was always so alarmed by the organs that I could barely look at them. If one were being played I would long to flee.

As a younger adult, before I had children and had time still to play the piano, I bashed out a few Bach fugues on the odd church organ, and once or twice in a cathedral, courtesy of a kind friend. I was always struck by the paradoxical relationship between the keys, stops and pedals. I often wondered how it was that the potential for the immeasurable multiplication of harmonies instilled in me not wonder but rather a fear of discordance. How Catherine got into playing one of those instruments regularly I do not know. There was certainly no religion involved at that point. I expect she simply enjoyed it.

I wanted to take a closer look at the musical instruments around the bed, to see if they were real or just toys, but in order to do so I had to stand on the bed. I tried very hard not to dislodge anything or disturb the bedclothes. Catherine was never coming back to them, I knew that, but she had been in them and not so long ago. They had covered her, kept her warm, and here I was treading on them. I began to question my self-imposed assignment. I asked myself whether I really should be there at all. Although Catherine had invited me, most often by phone, to visit her when she was alive, no plans of mine to do so had ever been followed through by her. I'd always had the feeling that she loved the idea but couldn't cope with the reality. If so, what right had I to be in her home now? Just our presence in the flat meant that we were standing on her things, and suddenly I felt as if we were violating everything that mattered to her. I told myself to get real. I told myself she would have walked over her own stuff all the time because there was no other way to get from *a* to *b* but I felt terrible standing on her bed. I got off it and apologised out loud.

'I'm sorry, Catherine,' I said quietly, feeling a little self-conscious. 'I'm not trying to hurt your home and I'm sorry I stood on your bed. I shouldn't have.'

That bed was probably where she spent a lot of her time, if not almost all of it, when she was at home. There was nowhere else to sit. I don't think she used the kitchen at all, or barely. It was tiny, situated in an alcove off the main room and cordoned off by a pair of pale yellow flowery curtains, drawn back and held in place by strings of wooden beads. To the right of the entrance was a circular mirror, to the left, fake flowers in a trio of hanging baskets. Within the kitchen were more pictures. On the fridge door, dolphins leapt from a dark blue moonlit sea. On the cupboard beside the fridge, ancient Egyptians stood in profile amongst hieroglyphs. Catherine's own versions of motorbikes, cars and parrots embellished the dirt-encrusted walls.

It looked as though she hadn't cooked for years. The cooker was mummified in layers of grime. So were the cupboards and so was the fridge. The fridge door was slightly ajar. Some theatrical-looking cobwebs, dark grey and withered, looped between the body of the fridge and its door.

I opened the door slightly. The cobwebs collapsed instantly and heavily. The fridge was empty.

I looked for a kettle and found a white plastic one. I vaguely remembered my mother mentioning that she'd found another one and thrown it out because – and this I now found comic in the extreme – it was broken. What difference the kettle's removal should have made I do not know. 'Why the kettle, Mummy?' I wanted to ask. Why on earth take one thing from this bedlam of expired articles? I almost laughed. I looked in the cupboards. A container of Pot Noodles. Some far-gone margarine. I don't know where Catherine ever got a proper meal.

I couldn't get her bed out of my head. I glanced across at it yet again and suddenly saw something on the window-ledge beyond it that I hadn't noticed before. It was a greetings card, the first that I'd yet seen. I picked my way back across the room and leant carefully across the bed to reach for it. The picture was of a blue sun with a face at its centre and blue rays radiating out from the face. It was cheerful and rather Eastern-looking. I picked it up and looked inside. It was from me. It was my response to an invitation from her to come and see her again. I had found the invitation the night I re-read all her letters to me. I had had no memory of it then, and it had devastated me, the thought that maybe I had failed to take her up on it.

Here it was, absolution, in my own writing. I had replied straight away to my sister. I had not abandoned her. I was so scared that I might have ignored her at a moment when she might have let me in but I hadn't done. Briefly I experienced the euphoria of vindication. She had obviously phoned me as well because I'd written, 'I'm so sorry I was out when you called, *please* phone me back to arrange a time for me to visit. I can't wait to see you.' I know she never did phone back because I know we never had that conversation.

I put the card in my coat pocket.

Stepping off the bed, I reflected upon it for a moment. Somehow, I couldn't bring myself to move the curled up sleeping-bag, there was something just too private about it, although I felt foolish leaving it as it was. So I straightened the blankets and cushions instead, leaving the teddy bear tucked up. I knew that anything I did was absurd because the next people to touch this bed would be those impenitents from the City Council, but it was hard not to pay even a little attention to the restoration of order. Now, the bed looked less like a lair even though it was a very long way from being inviting. I thought of tucking Clare into her cot and understood at that moment why my mother had jettisoned the broken kettle. It was a gesture of maternal care, futile but automatic. It's what mothers do. We tidy up. We try to make things nice for other people, even, so it seems, when the other people are dead.

In the corner of the room nearest the foot of Catherine's bed was what I took to be her Tibetan shrine. I went to look at it. In one of her letters, she'd told me about it. I'd sent her our wedding photograph and she'd written back to say how much she loved it, that she had put it on her shrine so she could look at it there in the candlelight. Now, there was no evidence of the photograph at all. On the wall above a makeshift altar were Catherine's own pictures of monks praying and monks surrounded by barbed wire, I assumed Chinese barbed wire.

Propped up against the wall behind the shrine were two large pieces of floppy, brown cardboard. She obviously used a lot of old stiff card and cardboard boxes on which to paint. Paper would have been far too expensive. Andrew had already found a lot of paintings done on the back of big display cards previously designed for use in shop windows. Catherine would have asked for these, probably. Despite her reclusive nature, she was never shy of asking for things. Both of the cards on the shrine had flopped over onto their faces, bendy with damp. Top Shop was written on the back of one. I turned it over.

'LIAR, LIAR,' it said.

I flipped over the second one.

'LIAR, LIAR,' it said.

This time, the words were underlined twice.

I turned my attention to the writing on the walls. Shivering, I had been unwilling to succumb to its power, had given myself over instead to the mighty disorder beneath my feet, but there was no avoiding it now.

T
  h
    a
      n
        k

          y
            o
              u

              G
                o
                d

T
h
a
n
k
s

S
i
r

N a n c i s d o y ! ! !
D u p c h a

This was all above the bed and there was a lot more like it besides. I didn't know if the words I did not recognise were Tibetan or not. Whatever the language, it made no sense to me. The words **STEFAN TIBET** were written beneath several pictures of fierce-looking Tibetans. The most prominent picture of all featured Stefan as a monk, imprisoned behind heavy steel gates held fast by a padlock emblazoned with a swastika.

I turned ninety degrees.

T h a n k   y o u   G e o r g e

I had no idea who George might be.

D r S t e v e n   S t e v e n z
S t e v e
S t e v e   d r   s t e v e n z
C I T Y

S t e v e   S t e v e . . . It was written everywhere, high and low, horizontal and vertical. Very often the name was followed by Catherine's address. Children do this when they learn to write; they write their names everywhere, and later, their addresses. They are staking their claim on themselves and their place in the world.

I turned another ninety degrees and noticed for the first time some large letters in between the footballing pictures. They were in vivid blue.

a n   s   f i

I removed two pictures from the wall to see where the letters belonged.

m e a n   w i t h   h i s   f i s t s

I stared at the words for a long time. Did they refer to anything specific, to anyone real? Was it just fantasy-induced paranoia or had some bastard punched my big sister? I would rather have been punched than see that statement.

I turned again, back to the Tibetan shrine, and there on the low patch of wall behind the Top Shop cards with their fierce accusations – **LIAR LIAR** - were the words:

L o r d   t h i s   c e l l   i s   c o l d

And in that cold cell I broke down and cried for a cold sister.

But there was loveliness, too. Interspersed between Catherine's own pictures were several, much larger, posters. Natural beauty was their theme. Mountains, seas, landscapes, animals, there was splendour and reverence in them all. The most imposing of them featured the black silhouette of a Hindu temple against a spectacular golden-orange sunset: *The Himalayas – A Shocking New Trek* stood out in gigantic white letters across the top. On its left was a painting of two majestic-looking stags in a snowy Scottish Highland landscape; on its right, an aerial photo of a tropical ocean at dusk, brushing gently against a deserted coastline. Beneath it was a painting of a galleon at sea. A circular sticker was stuck to the bottom right hand side of the painting: it said, *Peace.*

Catherine loved colour, it was obvious. Reds, oranges, yellows, greens, blues, purples: the full range was there, vivid and intense. For once, that tedious cliché 'a riot of colour' was apposite because there was indeed something riotous about the improbable blend of hues and tones. In their mixture was something tumultuous but magnificent, something wrong that managed, in those particular circumstances, to look appropriate.

Hanging from the walls at various angles were long strips of paper that had once entitled other posters: *Land of The Tiger; JAPAN; British Airways*. A partially obscured calendar displayed a photograph of a soldier in a beret: beneath the photo were the words, *The Light Infantry*. A fake coat of arms perched above a filthy and crumpled Union Jack, which in turn half-covered a picture of a cat decorated with gold and silver tinsel. Across all these posters and pictures sagged cobwebs so vast and baroque that they looked as if they had been carefully placed there to exaggerate a point about abandonment and decay.

All around the room were dozens of photographs of tigers, as well as calendars of African wildlife, bears and polar landscapes. A poster of a Spanish bullfighter in bloody conflict with a bull, and a white fur jacket hanging from the door to the main room, seemed at odds with Catherine's lifelong love of animals and her hatred of cruelty towards them. The jacket was especially bewildering. What spare money Catherine had had in the past she almost always felt compelled to give away, most often to charities that supported, rescued and protected animals. She belonged to the WSPA and RSPCA. She sent money to stop the fur trade, save the whale, train guide dogs for the blind; she sent it even as she was dying. It's possible that she had rescued the jacket, to save it from being worn.

Perhaps this was it. Perhaps all this before me was the evidence I had been seeking, evidence of a life lived outside. Maybe Catherine's engagement with the world was so much more obvious than I had at first thought when assaulted by this frenzy of information. The Himalayas, bears, dogs. Oppressed Tibetans. Football. Here was the outside world. Or rather, here was Catherine's outside world, there being no such thing as one outside world to which we can all relate, there being millions of people for whom Tibet, bears and football have no meaning, and upon whom they do not impinge in any way.

It was a world that Catherine clearly believed to be in need of change and improvement, a world that angered and upset her. Yet it was also a world in which she found things to enjoy, activities, sights and sounds that gave her pleasure. In all these ways, it was an outside world like most people's, a world governed by humanity's terrible misdemeanours but also by its sense of hope. Most important of all, it was an outside world containing others for whom Catherine had a measure of concern.

I don't know how you measure engagement with others, or even whether you should. Catherine engaged with other people at some distance: she engaged with races, causes or injustices but not individuals. This was probably the most possible, comfortable way for her to take an active social part in the world around her. I began to think that she lived her life as she was able, unselfconsciously and within her limits. Standing in what had been her home, I could no longer propose – as once I had – that she was 'cut off' from the outside world. She was in the world, she was part of it and she understood what it meant to her. And though I cannot know for sure, I don't think she felt herself defined by anything or anyone else. I doubt she thought of herself as blighted and unfortunate, in the way perhaps others thought of her. I doubt she thought very often of herself, really. Did she, then, know better than many the true taste of freedom?

I picked my way across to the window. It was in fact a full-length glass door that opened on to a balcony outside. There, on the balcony, was the only piece of furniture I had yet come across, an enormous armchair, low, deep-seated and sopping wet. Such a nice place for a chair and yet so hopeless. It had become a giant sponge. An enormous orange teddy bear was sitting on it. The teddy bear was drenched, too. I peered over the balcony, down to the flats' communal garden. Not bad, as these places go; it was tidy and well-kept, quite nicely designed. I could hear seagulls above my head and the raised soprano voices of young children playing nearby. I realised there was a primary school next door.

Back inside, I decided to take more photographs. I grew bold. I photographed the whole room, high and low, three hundred and sixty degrees. I spoke to Catherine as I did so. I asked for her permission. I said I knew she couldn't grant it but I hoped she didn't mind. I explained to her why I was doing it. I told her that I didn't want to forget where she'd lived and that I wanted a record of the home she had created. I know where and how my other siblings live. I know what their houses feel like and I recognise the clutter and comfort peculiar only to them. There are pieces of furniture from our family, our father's drawings on all our walls. Some of our photographs overlap. Our homes are like a dot-to-dot picture, they join up, related to one another not only by virtue of the people inside them but by the objects they contain.

It goes without saying that there was not a shred of evidence, except the card I had found, that Catherine had any family at all. But she did. She had me, for a start, right there in the room, cataloguing the past for the future. It's too bad, I thought: it's too bad if this annoys her. She was my sister and my daughter's aunt. I never disputed her right to disappear, none of us did, but I never disputed my right to care about her still. And now that imperative of duty and sorrow had led me here, with my plastic bags and my camera. After all, we were the ones who were left, not least with all her things. If most of them were destined for landfill, it was not she who would live with the decision. If her inheritance to us was that peculiarly ghastly judgment, then it was up to us how much was preserved.

So I took my photographs with ever-decreasing qualms and I told her ghost as much, if a ghost there was to witness my chronicling of a place in limbo, of a life elapsed.

What Is a Wardrobe?

When she left university, one of my best friends, Charlotte, went to live in a two-bedroomed flat in west London with a couple of her friends. Ali, an art student and the flat's owner, had the small bedroom to herself. Charlotte, who was training to be a primary school teacher, shared the bigger bedroom with Helen, a trainee lawyer. Either woman's visiting boyfriend meant the de-camping of that evening's lone spinster to the sitting-room sofa. The rest of the flat was a free-for-all, and I do not use the term lightly.

It was a household of glorious indulgence. Parties were frequent and impromptu. Boyfriends were steady but plenty of other people came and went at various and usually unspecified hours, cooking or consuming any available drinks and meals as they passed through. Shopping was shared and seemed to me, already at twenty-one a woman with a history of long, prissy shopping lists, entirely haphazard. There was sometimes enough food in the house, occasionally none (save some stale cream crackers and dried pasta), and when there was plenty it was prepared and served with relish. Domestically, I was appalled by the place. There was never enough space to wash up, the bathroom was furnished with damp bath towels, used coffee mugs, and tubes of Charlotte's lipstick and mascara at various stages of decay, and there was always noise from other people. But it was a perfectly wonderful place to be and I loved it. I hated the cigarette smoke but derived a huge, vicarious pleasure from all that it stood for, a kind of profound nonchalance about life that I have never had, often envied, but genuinely desired only fleetingly.

Nowhere was this nonchalance, this unplanned unfurling of each day, more apparent than in the lawlessness that was Charlotte's and Helen's wardrobe. The wardrobe was not a piece of furniture, nor a cupboard, nor a series of shelves, nor even a free-standing rail. The wardrobe was the entire bedroom floor. There's a refrain in a well-known children's story called *We're Going On A Bear Hunt*, which I read often to my daughters: when the family on said bear hunt encounter an obstacle on their journey – a river, snowstorm, or mud flat – up goes the chant, 'We can't go over it, we can't go under it. Oh no! We've got to go *through* it!' Well, Charlotte's and Helen's wardrobe was just like that. When getting dressed, wading was the better part of the procedure. And it was not just your average messy-person's room with stuff on the floor. It was much more as if a jumble sale had been shaken vigorously into the room from above. The impression was augmented by the fact that Charlotte and Helen slept on mattresses on the floor, under a soft miscellany of duvets and blanketry.

The clothes themselves were motley: short skirts, long skirts, little tops, big tops, baggy jerseys, trousers, shorts, blouses, sweatshirts, hats, scarves, jackets; every fabric, every colour; stripes, flowers, patterns, plain. There appeared to be no sense of ownership of the garments themselves, or almost none. Various items, if admired, were termed 'Charlie's' or 'Helen's' but that didn't prevent either one of the women wearing whatever she wished without the slightest reference to the other. Thus, the sense of a wardrobe not merely as a recognisable object but as a collection, an entity even, which suggested in visual terms a few basic facts about its owner, like choice, taste, occupation or even political sensibility, simply did not exist. At the very least, it was greatly undermined by Charlotte's and Helen's unconventional arrangement.

At Christmas-times, sharp with sorrow when I thought of my eldest sister, I would send her parcels of food or clothes. The last clothes I remember sending her were a large, warm fleece and some thick wool socks. I envisaged her chilly, clad in inadequate garments that were too lightweight for a cold English winter in a probably not well-heated council flat. I imagined her bony beneath thin denim jackets when what she needed, surely, was a soft jersey and thermal underwear. I thought of her eating tepid toast and cheap, pale biscuits while needing a serious mountain of a meal, steaming straight from the oven, announcing itself with fabulous scents and a blast of heat. On such imaginings, my guilt about my sister was sustained. While I thrived, she was under-dressed and undernourished.

The truth was rather different, at least as far as the clothes were concerned. On the immediate right of the front door to Catherine's flat was her bathroom. It had almost nothing to say for itself. Social Services had already been, I later learned, and stripped the bathroom and hallway of whatever stylistic resemblance they bore to the room in which Catherine lived, ate and slept. The bathroom paint was greying and the room was windowless, empty but for the bath, basin and loo. On the wall was a forlorn reminder that this room had once been Catherine's; a post card of the Himalayas and one of her own paintings of a tiger's face. But there was another room in the flat, to the right of the bathroom. There was another door, wedged open. I didn't notice it at first, I walked straight past it. Instead, fearful and fascinated, I was drawn to the room straight ahead, the one so strange and terrifying. But the other room was there all along like a coda to the first.

Its door was partially open. I pushed it gently, then harder. It wouldn't budge. Something was in the way. Rucked-up carpet? I couldn't really see. The daylight from the window in the room was compromised by something, which only added to the deep gloom, and it took my eyes a while to adjust. I put my head around the door to see what was in its way. Clothes. I shoved the door hard, discovered it wedged on both sides. The clothes had become stuck in the doorway. I squeezed past the door and into the tiny space between it and the jamb.

Wall to wall, with not an inch to spare, was a vast, heaving expanse of jackets, shirts, trousers, vests, ties, socks and jerseys. They were all men's. Strewn, tossed and tangled, the clothes' density and disposition suggested anger, confusion, possibly desperation, but certainly no kind of cheerful disregard. My God, I thought. My God. Because it wasn't just the breadth of the pile, it was the height, too. While Charlotte and Helen had successfully colonised every last inch of their bedroom floor, Catherine had gone up the walls, too. About four to five feet up, to be precise. The effect was nightmarish, an ocean in a bedroom.

The clothes themselves looked forsaken. In their evident uselessness they had assumed a strongly pathetic character, a personality even, as if they had been brought to Catherine's flat expecting so much more, expecting to be useful and possibly esteemed, but were instead now lying dead. Truly they looked as if some terrible violence had befallen them, as if the worst of Catherine's turbulence and confusion had culminated in their being cast off and discharged, not because they were surplus to requirements but because they were despised. If ever the haphazard disposition of material objects could suggest deep betrayal, they did.

It was impossible to know whether the garments' effect upon me had any basis in reality. It was hard to discern whether or not the pile's evolution lay in a kind of demented anger or just an unorthodox attitude to storage. But it was difficult to absorb whatever it may have represented without thinking of a discarded mass infinitely worse. An image came to me suddenly, an infamous image, of the broken bodies of the Jewish prisoners at Belsen. To draw any parallels between the results of Nazi evils and evidence of a sick woman's psychosis would be contemptible. Yet these material remains had a resonance all of their own, a resonance that reached beyond the immediate confines of their particular setting. That a pile of clothes could bring to mind such images of torment may illustrate only my particular comprehension of it, but it may also serve to underline the pile's intrinsic derangement.

In amongst the clothes, partially buried, but emerging at accidental angles, rather as if they were floating, were three tea chests. These were stuffed to the brims with more of Catherine's paintings. There were probably several hundreds in each, most of them on her trademark cardboard. I climbed onto the pile, which barely subsided under my weight, and started sifting through the tea chest nearest to the door. Here were more tigers, Tibetans, temples, motorbikes, flowers, and birds. I tried the second chest, which involved a further advance into the room. The same. I could see without climbing to the window that I didn't need to examine the third.

I contemplated the room. I tried to see it for what it was, not for what I thought it suggested. Catherine's wardrobe. Clearly, it was more than a statement about the tyranny of order. In fact, I doubt that it was any kind of statement at all. There is necessarily something rather public about a statement. A statement demands some kind of witness, a third party. Catherine's wardrobe, like Charlotte's and Helen's, was an expression, and a private, unselfconscious one at that. It wasn't for anyone, or anything. But what was it an expression of? I say I believe that Catherine's wardrobe suggested anger, confusion and desperation because, to me, that's what it looked like. When I see deep mess and disunity I see something wrong. And yet even that isn't quite right, or rather, it need not apply. After all, Charlotte's and Helen's wardrobe was evidence of a life in which having fun took precedence over all matters domestic, and as such it was an expression of happy, youthful neglect. But why was that obvious? Why would anyone looking at the two rooms know that Charlotte's and Helen's was acceptable and Catherine's was mad?

The lack of any pathway either into or through Catherine's room was a pretty fair indicator. There wasn't, strictly speaking, a pathway through Helen's and Charlotte's room either but you could have used the beds as stepping stones, and it was still possible to open the door. So is it a matter of scale? Why is it that ankle-deep clothes on a bedroom floor are okay, though probably only in the young, while piles four or five feet high are not, not even for anyone under twenty-five? When does mess stop being mess and become psychopathic disorder? Remembering the parcels of clothes I had sent to my sister, it was more than a little ironic to suppose that buried somewhere in that pile was the blue fleece I had been so convinced she needed. Had she lived to ninety, she would never have required it. Certainly, one could argue that Catherine didn't need half the clothes she had but was her hoarding of them in itself suggestive of a damaged personality? Millions of us hoard things and millions of people have far too many clothes.

So if the room was simply a wardrobe, what was wrong with it? People with the space and money have large wardrobes; some have dressing-rooms. Many of these are packed to the hilt, and not just with clothes. One of my wardrobes at home houses, amongst other miscellaneous objects, a baby crib, a cot mattress, some of my husband's many tennis racquets, and some rolled up floor rugs. Therefore, Catherine's joint storage of her pictures with her clothes was in keeping with tradition and neither odd nor surprising. However, while Catherine did not have ample space or quantities of money, and her lifestyle did not require a vast number of outfits, her clothes commandeered around a third of her living space. What's more, she would have had great difficulty locating most of them – assuming that that's what she wanted to do.

Surveying the room then, I couldn't believe that she did. Perhaps collecting things gave her pleasure. After all, it wasn't just clothes. The teddy bears, football paraphernalia, badges, clocks, tins, bags, shoes and radios across the hallway suggest that her impulse to collect – and alongside it, to hoard – found expression in all sorts of ways. Perhaps things simply interested her. Perhaps she thought they would come in handy one day. Perhaps they made her feel safe, or safer than contact with human beings. It may have been, when considering the agony and terror which was evident in the writing on the walls of Catherine's main room, that the many thousands of things in that same room provided comfort. Or perhaps she created the sort of disorder around her that was within her because, instinctively, that was how she understood the world.

Perhaps. Finding reasons for the degree of disarray in Catherine's physical environment doesn't quite answer the most important question that it poses. Does such confusion automatically point to madness? Most people would agree that the point at which it becomes enormously arduous and time-consuming to locate something you possess, not because it is lost but because your means of storage is impractical to the point of impossibility, is the point at which you and your method become inseparable. Personally, though, I'm not sure what this really means. If asked whether I would deem that room as being far from sane, I would not hesitate to say yes, but I would still be unable to describe how one can accurately measure something as non-specific and personal as mess. I do know that some people actually don't care about mess, and I have often wished I were one of them. I also know that things as mundane as laziness, lethargy or mild depression can prevent people from tidying up. People talk quite casually about things getting on top of them. For some, this phrase has genuine physical meaning. I wonder if at the heart of Catherine's pile existed the original challenge, something that was too difficult for her to tackle and therefore easier to bury.

A friend of mine called Alf, who lives alone in a remote tin-miner's cottage on the Cornish moors, co-exists quite happily with a houseful of broken irons, kettles, toasters, myriad tools, nuts, bolts, screws, and bits of ancient, anonymous metal. Some of the appliances belong to other people and most of them he's planning to repair, one day. Like Catherine did, Alf stays awake for much of the night, not because he's afraid of the dark but because he loves its peace. In the small hours, he listens to the BBC World Service and reads books about physics and engineering. Alf has a great sense of humour and a lot to say about politics. He is wonderfully, refreshingly unconventional but he certainly isn't crazy.

Alf claims to know exactly what he has in his house and where it is. Catherine might well have done the same, I don't know. So if disorder, scale and inconvenience do not account for the ultimate peculiarity of her wardrobe, is context necessary, too? Had Catherine been a straightforward hippie with an idle disrespect for traditional sartorial management, would her wardrobe have been quite as disturbing? It's hard to say but probably not. I knew she was ill and her wardrobe confirmed it. But were the specifics of her illness actually evident in it? Who is to say what size, and how organised, something has to be in order for it to make sense? I once knew an elderly woman who kept paper bags, obsessively. They covered her kitchen table, rendering it absolutely useless, and the pile was taller than she was. Being light, the bags zig-zagged onto the floor whenever there was a draught, which effectively meant every time someone opened the kitchen door. But because she was a language scholar with a sharp wit she was regarded as bright and eccentric, no more, no less. She was actually rather unpleasant but that isn't relevant. Being a pain in the neck doesn't make you a nutter.

I can only conclude that, as in so many other things, it is a question of entirety. Catherine's wardrobe alone is bizarre but unclear. But the wardrobe as a close relative of her living room and a product of her actions and choices; the wardrobe as an indicator of her broken personality; the wardrobe as an outward expression, or symbol, of internal fragmentation; the wardrobe as a rejection of feminine tastes and the confirmation of Steve's presence in Catherine's life; that wardrobe has much to say for its owner, its creator.

A collection of clothes. A repository for the personality.
What is a wardrobe?

Weird Things That Happened, One: Catherine's Will

And that should have been it. It was enough, after all, just being in that place which raised more questions than it answered. That should have been the end of the search.

But it wasn't. Andrew was rooting around in the room full of clothes, his arms plunged deep into the mass of garments. He wasn't having a great deal of success finding anything but more and more clothes and more and more pictures. And then, from the subterranean depths of clothes, pictures and wallpaper sample books, where material and papers were both tangled and tightly packed, their fusion so dense that in places they were set like concrete, he pulled out a large piece of greyish brown card. It was very like the one on which _LIAR_, _LIAR_ was written.

I had my head in one of the tea chests full of pictures but in my peripheral vision I saw him pull it out and I heard him exhale.

'Mary, look at this.'

'What?'

'Look.' He held out the card.

'What is it?'

'Just have a look.'

I took the card. It was plain on one side. I turned it over.

Please give me a church funeral

I turned it over and then back again.

Please give me a church funeral.

I clambered back over the pile and into the hall. I placed the card on the pile of pictures I had selected to take away from the flat. I didn't say a word. Neither of us did.

Until, some moments later, I said, 'You have to be kidding.'

Andrew said, 'Damn right.'

'To find that,' I said, 'I mean, of all the things in here.'

'I know.'

I shook my head, full of sorrow. Here was a written request of such clarity. It was so spare, so unfettered. I don't know when Catherine wrote it or in what state. I don't know to whom it was intended, if anyone, and whether she'd intended it to be found or just written it on the spur of the moment. I don't know whether it was written in a moment of madness or one of lucidity. And I don't know if it was meant for us at that moment because I don't know whether spirits exist, and if they do, whether they have any part to play in our lives. What I do know is that it was one of the saddest things I had ever seen.

I looked at my husband.

'Are you freaked out?'

He thought for a moment.

'Not really,' he answered.

'Not really?'

'Well,' he conceded, 'maybe a bit, yes.'

'I am,' I said.

I was. I felt cold all over.

He said, 'Don't tell your folks.'

I said, 'I don't know.'

He said, 'Don't, darling. It won't help.'

*   *   *

We went downstairs to let Steve Shepherd know that we were done. As he was locking up he said, 'I'm very sorry about Cathy. It's very sad.'

'Did you have much to do with her, Steve?' I asked.

'No. To be honest, you know, she always kept herself to herself.'

'Did she get on with the other people in the building?'

He shrugged slightly.

'She acknowledged them, she acknowledged me. Sometimes she'd stop and chat and sometimes she'd just acknowledge you and then go on her merry way.'

Merry. Did Catherine have a merry way? Was 'merry' a word that related to her, really?

I told Steve about the two men from the Council.

'Yeah, they really shouldn't have turned up,' he said. 'It's very odd that they came because I haven't sent the letter off yet. Your mum signed a letter authorising us to get the flat cleared but I haven't sent it on to the Council yet. I can't understand why they've come.'

'Well, if they'd come to clear another flat, maybe they thought they could clear this one at the same time.'

'Yes, but they didn't know it needed clearing. It doesn't make any sense.'

I didn't know what to say. He was right. It didn't make sense.

Steve asked me what I wanted to do.

I said, 'Well, it's not up to me. I'll have to ask my parents and they'll let you know. Is that okay?'

'Of course.'

'Probably it's fine for the Council to go ahead on Monday but I don't know if anyone else wants to come back down here.'

I knew I didn't want to. I never wanted to see that flat again.

'Sure,' said Steve. 'No problem.'

He was looking at me sideways.

'I can see Cathy in you,' he said.

Andrew and I loaded what we'd taken of Catherine's things into the boot of the car. Everything was in bin-liners. We'd sorted through it all wearing rubber gloves because of the dust. My mother had said, 'Take rubber gloves,' and I'd taken one pair for me and none for Andrew because I knew he wouldn't wear them. But in the end I'd persuaded him, with difficulty, to squeeze a hand into one of mine.

'Oh, come on,' he'd complained. 'I can't wear rubber gloves. For God's sake, darling, how many men do you know who wear rubber gloves?'

'This is an unreal situation.'

'You can say that again.'

I had despised myself for wearing those gloves. As I'd sorted through Catherine's possessions, I'd thought, This is my sister, her home, her life, and I'm handling what is left of it all with rubber gloves. How revolting of me. Why can't I just handle her things properly? But there were practical reasons why not. I had the baby and there was no way of cleaning up afterwards. There was water in the flat but it was cold and there was no soap, I hadn't thought to bring some. I had to handle Clare, had to feed her. I couldn't feed a small baby covered in a film of dirt and decay.

'I'm filthy,' I said, when we'd finished.

'We can go to that shop I've just been to,' Andrew suggested, 'and have a cup of tea in the café there while you feed Clare. There are loos there.'

The prospect of tea and soap was enticing.

'Good idea.'

From around the corner of the building the two Council workers reappeared. I hoped they wouldn't see us, or at least, if they did that they wouldn't approach us.

The shorter one came and stood right next to me. I could practically feel him breathing.

'Sorry about that,' he said, too loudly. 'It's just, you know, we had instructions to clear the flat.'

'That's fine,' I said, 'don't worry about it.'

'Oh well, you know, hope we didn't cause offence.'

'Listen, it's fine. It doesn't matter.'

'We had instructions, you see.'

I tried a bit of gallows humour.

Indicating the building, I said, 'Well, you've got your work cut out up there.'

'Oh no,' he countered. 'I've seen worse than that. I've had them up to here.' He gestured with his right hand flat under his chin. 'That's nothing.'

'Oh. Right.'

But they didn't leave. This man was bent on making what he believed to be an apology for having turned up. He told us how the flat just had to be cleared. How no-one had told them they couldn't do it. How they had to get it done because of the new tenant coming. I didn't ask him where his information had come from. I shut out his voice and my mind wandered to one of my nephews, an athletic teenager who once endearingly referred to mountain biking as his 'premier sport'. 'Apology,' I wanted to say to the man, 'is not your premier social skill.'

'So,' he was saying, 'it wasn't like we had any choice.'

'I know that,' I replied, though none of it made any sense. 'I understand.'

'We have to get these things done. We can't hang around.'

'I know, I understand you're just doing your job.'

'There's someone new coming, you see.'

'Yes.'

Someone new. Maybe it would be someone with altogether different problems. Maybe it would be someone who would leave the re-painted magnolia walls bare, who would have pot plants and a sofa.

Andrew decided he had had enough and managed, adroitly and swiftly, to get rid of the two men. I looked up at the sky, which was charcoal with rain clouds, until I was sure they had gone.

They had gone. Andrew was laughing.

'They were pretty funny,' I agreed.

He said, 'There was something Shakespearian about the way they kept appearing.'

'How do you mean?'

'Gravediggers,' he said.

My uncle was a photographer. Shortly before he died, Andrew and I visited him and asked to look through some of his photographs. He had thousands, beautifully archived. I remember that day being struck as never before by the fact that the act of looking at a photograph places you in the shoes of another person more directly than any other medium. As I looked at a collection of photos of sunlit rivers and hot French streets, my uncle said, 'I was about fifteen when I took those.'

I thought, I'm standing where you stood: this is remarkable.

A boy in short trousers appeared in the next photograph, in the middle distance.

'Who's that?' I asked.

'Your father,' said my uncle.

On returning to the car after our trip to the DIY store café, I saw from a different angle the building in which Catherine had lived.

I wondered how often she had turned the corner we had just turned. I wondered if her feet had been on precisely the patch of ground that mine were on now.

I'm standing where you stood.

'I want to photograph the outside,' I said to Andrew. 'I won't be a minute.'

I took some photographs. Then I positioned myself before the main entrance door to the building. Catherine would have opened this door whenever she went out, and when she came back from wherever she'd been this is exactly where she will have stood. I lifted my hand to touch the door handle. It was predictably cold and hard. It gave up nothing of my sister. I thought then, How crazy and strange is our investment of everyday objects with sacred meaning.

Driving away from the flat through Clifton, which is one of Bristol's plushier areas, I looked at all the smart shops, brightly lit. How did she feel about shops like this, selling expensive cappuccino and baguettes, pretty and pointless gifts, well-cut clothes? It was impossible to know. I looked out of the car window while we waited at some traffic lights and I took in a tapas bar, a delicatessen, a wine bar, a fancy sandwich shop, an art gallery, a Japanese restaurant.

Was all this part of her world? If so, was it any more than a view? I don't know how much she looked around her and what she saw when she did. What did she make of places like these? Did she see these boutiques, galleries and restaurants as places she couldn't afford to go into? Did she desire the goods inside? Were they places she went to for conversation, change, an escape from bad weather? Or were these emporia chiefly sources of colour and light? A shop is like a wardrobe, I began to think, a place that begs a question.

Andrew and I talked a lot of the way home. We were both shocked by what we'd seen and felt. Andrew said that when he was in the kitchen, he hadn't liked standing with his back to the main room. I said I'd felt much the same. We agreed we'd both felt watched. We agreed we'd felt Catherine was there. We agreed that it was probably all conjecture and unease on our parts, no more or less than a mixture of fear and imagination.

In the back of the car was our baby daughter, sleeping, luminously beautiful. In the boot was Catherine's stuff, a fraction of it. Three bin liners, a flat stack of paintings and the card: *Please give me a church funeral.* Catherine's only known will.

I sighed deeply, spent by a day that had begun in the morgue where Catherine lay dead and ended in the flat where she had lived. I was inebriated by too much information and too many people: Mr Carpenter and the nurses; Jo Fleming, Steve Shepherd and the gravediggers. Steve Stevenz.

L o r d   t h i s   c e l l   i s   c o l d

Andrew patted my thigh.

'Get some sleep, darling,' he said, gently.

I closed my eyes. He flicked on some soft jazz; Dave Brubeck, *Take Five.* The music drifted in and out of me as the car hummed steadily along the motorway into a blackened night.

Weird Things That Happened, Two: The Vanishing

I didn't show the ragged grey card to my parents but of course I told them what was written upon it. How could I not?

'Please give me a church funeral,' I reported, the words smaller in my mouth than they had been on the card.

We were in my parents' kitchen. My father had just made himself a cup of coffee. He absorbed the information and left for his own room and his work, aiming for the sanctuary of a place where there wasn't going to be a drawn-out conversation between women.

My mother said, through springing tears and gritted teeth, 'Well then, she shall have it.' She said it with ferocity, as if it were something she would do for Catherine even if the request were not straightforward, even if it were something for which she had to walk over hot coals.

And when she nearly cried, my beautiful, brave mother, I hugged her and said, 'Mummy, this is good. At least we all know what she wants, we know what to do.'

We drank tea and looked at the photographs of my recent skiing holiday with Andrew and Clare. The pictures were all of the baby: we could have been anywhere.

'Catherine was a good skier,' my mother remarked, in matter of fact tones.

'Was she? I never realised that.'

'She was terribly athletic,' my mother continued. 'She was the fastest runner of you all, by a long way.'

I knew that. I remembered being envious of her speed when we chased each other around the orchard. She was one of those people you could never, ever catch. I also remembered Catherine's facility for twisting her body into bendy yoga poses. I could see her now, sitting for what seemed like hours in the lotus position in her bedroom or on the lawn, eyes closed, prayer beads dripping from her wrist. She taught me to sit in the lotus position, side by side with her. Though I could never maintain a pose as she could, I stayed still for as long as possible in a small girl's homage to the strange and riveting romanticism of an older sister. Her legs were long and strong, her hands like a boy's, her face unadorned.

'How tall was she?' I asked my mother, my mind on Catherine's wonderful limbs.

'I don't know,' said my mother. 'Fairly tall.'

'But how tall? She was taller than I am, right?'

My mother thought about this. 'I'm not certain she was, actually. I'd say she was a little shorter than you.'

'No. Surely not.'

I had memories of Catherine's impressive height but then I was only little when she was big. And what I remember from my own teens and early adulthood had much more to do with what might be going on inside her head than whether or not that head was a couple of inches or so above my own.

'Let's see,' said my mother, getting up from the kitchen table to look behind the kitchen door. Behind the kitchen door is the place on the wall where all our childish heights are marked. New Year's Day was traditionally the day for measurement, though nobody ever remembered, and years came and went without record of one or another of us. It's a patchy, arbitrary chronicle and although the area on which it is documented is a protected zone, a couple of measurements disappeared accidentally under a layer or two of paint one year. Still, for all its lack of integrity it manages to reflect some truth about our growth as a family.

It reflects something else, too. As I perused the wall, I thought that despite her grief my mother was none the less a fortunate woman, for you can do this sort of thing if you plan never to move house; you can chart your growing brood behind the kitchen door with certainty. You know you can refer to a strip of yellowing plaster for information if your children have stood – and your grandchildren still stand – with their backs straight and their heels against the same bit of skirting board. I think that wall reveals more about my family than our relative sizes. I suspect what it really discloses is what we assumed about our place in the world as we grew up. Its more telling record may be that of a certain sort of privilege. My mother did not expect to move house, not because she and my father did not expect to progress through life but because the whole notion of progress would never have occurred to them. By the time they were in their late twenties, with three children under the roof of their beautiful home, they were already in place. In more ways than one they were where they had always assumed they would be and intended to stay. The height chart said it all. Only a mother with complete confidence in the solidity and immutability of her family life would embark upon such a precious record in a place that cannot be removed.

I looked at my own first measurement: MMBL – Jan '67.

'How did you manage to do that?' I asked, 'I was only six weeks old then.'

'I can't remember,' my mother answered. 'I think we probably measured you with a tape measure and then put the measurement on the wall.'

I looked for Catherine's initials. CML. I remembered that one of her measurements stuck out slightly to the right. CML – '72, I think; the year before her most catastrophic breakdown.

My mother looked, too. We peered in silence, up and down the wall.

'I can't see them,' I said.

My mother wrinkled her nose and frowned over the top of her glasses.

'I can't see them either. How odd.'

'They must be there,' I said.

'Well,' said my mother, 'you'd have thought so.'

We continued to search.

I protested, 'They can't not be here. They can't have just vanished.'

But they had.

'I suppose they might have been painted over,' said my mother. 'It's quite possible.'

'They can't have been,' I said, 'not all of them. She appeared several times. And the 1972 one was round about here – ' I pointed to the wall where my sister's measurement was not – 'sticking out slightly. I know it was because it was prominent and I used to notice it occasionally. And it can't have been painted over because look, there's one here done in 1971 for one of the others and it sticks out further than all of them, and that hasn't been painted over.'

My mother was still looking.

'And anyway,' I persisted, 'like I said, she appeared more than once. All her initials can't just have gone.'

But they had. As ever, Catherine was proving impossible to pin down. Still, this was taking even her most extreme hermitude into quite another sphere.

'Well,' said my mother, 'how very odd.' But she said it calmly, as if it made some sense to her. 'It looks as if Catherine has removed herself.'

I stared at her.

'You can't really think that.'

I was close to thinking it myself but I was awe-struck by my mother's application of her familiar rationale.

'Can't I?' she replied. 'Okay, I haven't the faintest idea what's happened but I know she's not there. Like you, I thought she was.'

I looked at the strip of wall devoid of the initials CML and any hint of where those initials might have been, and I backtracked.

'She must have been painted over that time,' I said, conceding to something approaching reason.

'Hmm,' said my mother, not conceding to it.

We returned to the table and our cooling tea and agreed that it was more than faintly bizarre.

Then I got up and looked at the wall again, convinced we must have missed something. We hadn't. There was still nothing.

'You really think she's removed herself, don't you,' I said.

So much for the permanence of our family record. That all evidence of Catherine appeared to have been impermanent was not only beyond comprehension, it was beyond irony.

'I don't know,' my mother replied. 'I simply don't know.'

'And you don't mind not knowing,' I said. It was a statement, not a question.

'Well, I do mind her not being there,' my mother replied. 'But I don't mind not knowing why because minding is neither here nor there.'

'How do you mean it's neither here nor there?'

'Minding,' she said, 'is not relevant.'

She was right, of course, my mother who is robust and truthful always. Even at her most troubled, even in pain, she embraces uncertainty when others might seek explanation.

She accepts mystery, if not without question then without any expectation of an explanation where none is necessary or sufficient. If she appeared indomitable when faced with perhaps the most decisive of Catherine's disappearances, and this one post-mortem as well, it was not because she did not care or was not perplexed. It was because she is someone who properly understands two of life's fundamental precepts: that uncertainty is to be expected and minding is not relevant. And therein lies her strength.

Funeral

Some things should go to the grave.
Catherine's funeral is one of them.

PART TWO: MIDDLE

Afterwards

Afterwards, there were two things I could have done with all the questions that were left in Catherine's wake: ignore them, or try to find some answers.

'You could talk to Karen Ainsley,' said Steve Shepherd, the caretaker, when I asked him about anyone who might have known my sister. 'She might know. Karen's worked in the building here for seven years.'

'What does she do?'

'She's a care worker. There are two of them here.'

He gave me Karen's telephone number. He also told me that Catherine used to visit a nun. He didn't know where the nun lived. He had a vague idea that her name might be Margaret but he couldn't swear to it.

When Catherine failed to meet her grocery bill, she would ask the owner of the local shop to send the bill to her mother. This he did, and our mother would pay. She still had the address and telephone number of the shop's owner, and his name, George Jefferies.

While Catherine's obsession with Buddhism never waned, during her late twenties some of her energy translated itself into something different and she was officially prepared for and received into the Roman Catholic Church. I remembered our parents being hopeful that it would bring some stability and peace to her life. I was surprised by their reaction. We were a strictly non-religious family, after all. But I have children now and so I understand. I know what hope my parents must have invested in anything legal that seemed to make their eldest daughter happy, or happier.

I figured that if Catherine went to church it was probably not a great distance from her home. I reasoned that wherever it was, there would be a finite number of Roman Catholic churches in Bristol.

I began with the nun who may have been called Margaret. If I'd thought about locating one woman in a city of nearly 400,000 people, I might have started with someone else. I might have started with Karen Ainsley or George Jefferies. They had names already. But I didn't start with them. Nuns tend, after all, to live in religious communities, which narrows it down. Anyway, my first book was about nuns and I decided that if anyone should be able to find one, I should. I think I also thought that I should start with something tricky. I don't know why. Perhaps the little bit of me that was still alive to thrill in those raw days following the funeral enjoyed the prospect of a challenge.

I rang someone I knew who worked for the Catholic Media Office and asked him for the names and telephone numbers of some Roman Catholic religious orders in Bristol. I began with the *Sisters of Charity*. Those Sisters didn't know my sister. I moved on to the *Sisters of Mercy*, then to *Our Lady of The Mission*, then the *Little Sisters of The Poor*. There were some Sister Margarets among them but not one was able to help. I tried the *Sisters of The Holy Cross* and the *Sisters of the Sacred Heart*. To a woman, they wished me well and asked God to bless me in my search but no one had heard of either Catherine or Stevie. Though I tried several times, I couldn't get a reply from the *Sisters of Saint Joseph*, so I left a message.

Next, I tried some Roman Catholic presbyteries in the hope of finding the church that Catherine may have visited. *The Church of Our Lady of Lourdes and Bernadette. The Church of the Holy Cross. St Nicholas's. St Patrick's. St Mary on the Quay. Christ The King. St John Fisher. Sacred Heart.*

Nothing.

Dispirited, I moved on to where I probably should have begun: George Jefferies, the man who owned and ran the grocery store where Catherine shopped. He was delighted to hear from me. I was amazed. For some reason, I had thought he might put the phone down on me.

'Do you think it might be possible to meet?' I asked him, nervously.

'With pleasure,' said George. 'Of course.'

I told him that I was looking for the church Catherine went to.

'I'm pretty sure,' said George, 'she went to the one next door to this shop.'

The church next door was St Nicholas of Tolentino. The priest's name was Richard McKay.

A week after leaving a message for him, Richard McKay phoned me back, full of apology. He'd been away on holiday.

He had indeed known Stevie. And he would be more than happy to meet me, any time that suited.

Beethoven on Platform One

Perched on the edge of her chair, Karen Ainsley shivered and held on to her foam cup of tea. She was probably as cold as I was.

It had seemed like a good idea at the time. We had planned to meet in the café on platform one of Bristol Temple Meads Station. The station was close to Karen's office but not in it: in it we might be disturbed and anyway, I had no wish to return to the building where Catherine had lived, and Karen's office was in that building.

However, when I arrived, the station café was closed. It wasn't going to open either, not this morning and not this month by the look of it. It was being dismantled and refurbished. Bang went my plans for a second breakfast. Attached to high scaffolding were giant plastic tarpaulin sheets. They flapped in angry gusts of wind, a bitter wind that forced its way along the open lines and into the station's vast and cavernous space in which, newly confined, it tussled with itself.

My hair whipped around my neck and face. It was about two degrees centigrade, disregarding the negative effects of wind chill. Irate, I swore and looked around. There were benches to sit on and there was a drinks vending machine planted near one of the benches. It was clearly temporary, put there while the café was out of commission, but it felt like a personal insult to me, a perfectly placed rebuke to someone with altogether different ideas about the provenance of a hot drink. Why, I asked myself, am I about to spend the morning frozen and hungry in pursuit of my dead sister when I could be tucked up at home reading *Field Mouse House* to my daughter?

I knew why, really.

Karen Ainsley was a nice-looking woman of about my own age, with glossy brown hair. Dressed in a pretty skirt, knee-high boots and a shapely jacket that implied that she cared about the cut of her clothes, she looked to me like an attractive primary-school teacher. She was carrying a large shoulder bag, bulging with papers.

When she arrived she apologised for being late.

I said, 'You're not late at all but we do have a slight problem.'

I indicated the café.

'Oh no,' said Karen.

'I think we're stuffed,' I said, and I pointed out the vending machine. 'That's our only option, unless you know anywhere nearby.'

'I don't,' said Karen, 'there isn't anywhere, not nearby anyway. I guess we'd better sit down there.'

She pointed at a single steel, circular table that I hadn't previously noticed. Cast adrift from the immediate environs of the dismantled café it was stranded on the other side of the vending machine. There were three chairs around it.

'If that's okay with you,' she added.

'Sure,' I said. 'It's fine. No worries.'

So we sat there together, drinking tea and stiffening with cold, while Karen outlined her role in Catherine's life. She was not a social worker but her background was in voluntary housing organisations and she was paid by the City Council. She worked alongside one other person from an office on the ground floor of the flats where Catherine had lived. Their approach was softly-softly.

'What we have in the building,' she explained, 'is called "low level supported housing", so we've a mix of people living there. There are people with mental health problems, people that have alcohol and drug misuse problems, people with learning difficulties, physical disabilities. And I suppose the crux of our role is to help people maintain their tenancies in the community, because some people might go in and out of psychiatric hospital while others may have been in hospital but now need a little bit of support just to carry on living independently.'

'And you're there as a supporting presence?'

'Yes,' said Karen, 'and the way that we work at the flats, we wait for people to come to us, we have an open door.'

I wondered whether Catherine walked through that open door much. I couldn't really imagine so. I thought of her own open doors, the ones inside the flat, jammed into position by clothes, tins, shoes, paints and boxes.

'But do you ever initiate contact?' I asked.

Karen shook her head, firmly.

'We don't check up on people,' she replied, 'unless we're concerned about their welfare. We wait for people to come to us because over the years we've found that that works. That's how people feel comfortable, coming in when they've got a letter they don't understand or they want to have a chat about something.'

'I see.'

An announcer's voice burst from the station tannoy system:

'*The train now approaching platform thirteen is the ten twenty-six for London Paddington, calling at Bath Spa, Chippenham, Swindon, Didcot Parkway, Reading, Slough and London Paddington. The train now approaching platform thirteen is the ten twenty-six for London Paddington.'*

'Did Cathy use you at all?' I asked, once the noise had subsided.

'Very seldom.' Karen shook her head. 'Very seldom. I mean, she was a very private person, she kept very much to herself. But she seemed to use me if she had letters that she wanted to write.'

'Letters?'

'Yes,' said Karen. 'In particular, she kept saying that she wanted to write letters to Amnesty International, and I don't know whether she did but she'd come in and check whether she had the right address and if I could write it on an envelope for her. Sometimes she'd get a bit agitated but then she'd calm down again quite quickly. It would be a momentary thing when she first came in to the office: "I need to write to Amnesty International and I need to do it today." And I'd say, "Right, okay, let's get the address," and she'd calm down.'

'Did she say why she was writing?'

'No, she didn't.'

A train exploded into the station like a fury and shot out the other side.

'More tea?' I offered.

'Yeah, thanks, that'd be lovely.'

I returned from the vending machine balancing two over-full cups.

'When I first started there,' Karen continued, 'she would bring some of her paintings in for me and maybe have a two-minute chat and then disappear again. That was what her contact was like. I think she felt comfortable just knowing that somebody was there.'

I began to enquire of Karen what Catherine talked about when she came in to the office but was interrupted by the arrival of the delayed service for Plymouth.

'*We are sorry,*' said the station announcer, '*for any inconvenience this has caused.*'

'A lot of times,' said Karen, cradling her cup in her hands, 'it was about Tibet and the monks, and I remember having a couple of discussions on Buddhism and what I felt about Buddhism. She asked me, did I know much about it? And I didn't know much, to be honest. I also didn't know anything about her background, what her life experiences had been up to when she moved into the flat. I didn't know whether she was a Buddhist or whether that was just an interest.'

'I think it was an interest,' I said, realising that I might more accurately have described it as an obsession, 'but an enduring one. It had lasted since she was in India in her early twenties. She never actually went to Tibet itself.'

'Right,' said Karen. 'Now I think about it, her conversation was mostly about the monks. It was almost as if she was in awe of them, not frightened exactly but there was definitely something she didn't like about them.'

Catherine had always talked and written so rapturously about Tibetan monks that I was a little startled by that. To seek spiritual enlightenment as a Tibetan monk represented for Catherine the greatest of all possible earthly achievements, or at least that's what I had thought. Yet it was true that there was a strong underlying menace in many of the paintings of those monks that I'd found at the flat. I had assumed that the violence etched into their faces was symbolic of the agonies they suffered under the Chinese regime. It seemed now that it might have indicated something else.

'How do you mean?' I asked.

'Well,' said Karen, 'she seemed to be in conflict over what she felt about them, or that's how it struck me. She was in awe of the way they lived their lives, of their solitude and how they devoted their lives to living that way. On the other hand, she implied that there were things they do that they shouldn't and that was never elaborated on. I don't know what that was because the conversation was always cut off at that point. There was something she didn't like about them but she wasn't going to expand on it.'

'Was she ever aggressive herself?' I asked, thinking to myself, She used to be. She used to frighten people.

'I've never seen her aggressive,' said Karen. 'We would quite often pass on the street and she'd tell me a joke and then walk away again. She always seemed quite happy within herself in that way. As I say, she was very private, so it was quite hard to get to know her completely, but I think she was happy and she seemed to me quite a gentle person.'

Gentle. Gentle could easily be a kind word used to describe someone silent and withdrawn. Was gentle exactly what Karen meant, or did she mean instead that my sister was sad?

'I wouldn't have said she was a sad person,' Karen replied. 'But I always had a feeling that something sad had happened to her. Obviously, she was very, very ill but I would have said she was happy within herself.'

I'm not sure that I would have said the same thing, having seen her flat. But then I didn't really know, did I. I had only the detritus of a life to sift through. Karen had seen Catherine regularly, in the flesh. Would she have felt differently if she had been inside Catherine's flat, to that terrifying inner sanctum? Perhaps she had been in, after Catherine died. And when considering Catherine's general state, did she discount all the evidence of a mind gone wild and accept her purely as she found her? Or did she believe that Catherine was cheerful, contented even, despite her illness?

Insanity, even fleeting insanity, looks like such a terrible thing when observed from the outside. The potency of psychosis makes it hard to believe that anyone burdened with it can be happy. Yet we all understand that happiness is relative. We learn to bargain with the world almost as soon as we enter it, developing ways of surviving by subdividing our attentions: we have words for disappointment, cruelty and destruction but we still smile. We live contentedly even though we are permanently compromised by our knowledge of the world. Is it a form of collective insanity, then, that we are able to rejoice despite our global calamities? People die unfulfilled and glaciers melt but birthday parties are still thrown and the sun shines on a billion gardens. Are we crazy to enjoy these things? Karen thought Catherine reasonably happy within herself. That goes for most of us. We are, to some extent, reasonably happy within ourselves despite the horrors. Does that make us mad, too?

I asked Karen, 'Did you never go into the flat in the time that you knew Catherine?'

'No,' said Karen. 'Oh no. Unless we're concerned for somebody's wellbeing or safety we won't go in. She invited me into the hallway a couple of times and I could see through the glass if I put notes or letters through her door. I could see quite obviously the way that she lived - I mean, the way she chose to live,' she corrected herself, 'but I only ever went into the hallway. She never invited me in. She was happy to let repair people in but it was very much, "This is my space."'

I said, 'I understand.'

'You could see that she kept things,' Karen said, a little hesitantly, 'in quite a chaotic manner. But as far as I was aware it didn't seem to be something that would impinge on her personal safety or health. There were obviously clothes left around and her pictures, but there weren't bags of rubbish and so I never felt any reason to go in.'

Reasons and non-reasons. Respect and interference. I was familiar with those particular dilemmas. I could see Karen's point exactly, and I approved of non-intervention, but I was still unclear how and where people such as she drew the line, professionally speaking. Perhaps there weren't bags of rubbish in Catherine's home but even discounting the scale and style of 'the way she chose to live' there was a defunct, cobweb-covered fridge, cooker and heater, and a broken kettle. And I have no idea what the bathroom was like before Social Services had had a go at it, in the final few weeks of Catherine's life.

'I did wonder,' I said, carefully, 'because when I saw the flat I wasn't aware of what your role was.'

'Right, yeah.'

'And I'm very well aware that she would have been quite jealous of her space.'

'Yes.'

'And also, I'm sure if someone had said, "Do you want a new cooker?" or "Do you think this needs a bit of tidying?", she probably would have told them where to go.'

Karen said, emphatically, 'Oh, definitely.'

'But I wasn't sure,' I continued, 'if your role is one where you try to make suggestions or whether your role is different. And I'm now realising it's different.'

'Yes,' said Karen. 'We didn't interfere. I was aware that she used to use the cafés locally, so we knew that she was eating. She always looked physically well so we knew that she wasn't neglecting her personal hygiene or well-being. She was always very slim but I think that was part of her build anyway.'

'It was,' I said. 'Do you happen to know which cafés she went to?'

'I saw her using two or three,' Karen replied. 'I don't know if there was a regular one.'

'I'd like to go and see them if I can.'

I had a fantasy about eating where she had. Perhaps I would sit where she once sat, watching the world from her table. It was as close as I would get to a meal with my sister. I couldn't remember the last one I'd had with her, apart from tea at the flat with the Michael Jackson montage. Was it breakfast, lunch or supper? I hadn't the ghost of a notion.

'Yeah, well I remember one was Barry's Café,' Karen said. 'I can explain to you where it is. The other place that I know she used to use was the Methodist Centre near here. It's around the corner from Barry's and it runs various groups for homeless people but they do accept other people. A lot of the time it does lunches, it's a drop-in for people to meet, to go and have a chat. They have clothing in there too, and laundry facilities.'

I watched a piece of loose newspaper dance maniacally up platform two. I felt suddenly enervated at the thought of drop-in centres, passed-on clothes and communal washing-machines. It seemed so depressing.

'You know,' said Karen quietly, sensing my dip in mood, 'she'd made the choices that she did and she was happy with those. I mean, she did go into hospital a couple of times over the last few years but it was only for very short periods of time and I think she herself noticed when she was ill. I know that her GP had her admitted but the impression I had was that each time she went into hospital she actually approached the GP herself first and asked to go in.'

'I see.'

I would have to write to Jo Fleming. There was so much that probably only she knew. I had been thinking about her a lot but I hadn't yet had the courage to do anything.

'I would imagine that she went in under a Voluntary Section,' Karen continued, 'which you can do for up to twenty-eight days. If you do that, you then have the right to leave when you want to. Quite a lot of people will go in under the twenty-eight-day Voluntary Section because if they feel a bit better and they don't want to stay in hospital for the full time, they don't have to.'

'Right.'

The station announcer cut across us once more.

'Did you know,' I asked, afterwards, 'that she was living as Stevie?'

'Yeah.'

'Did you know her as Cathy first?'

'Yes, I did. I knew her as Cathy because when I started the post I had a list of names and details of everybody in the flats. The first time that she came down to see me I used the name Cathy and she corrected me. She said, "Actually, my name's not Cathy." But I do know that on a couple of notes I absent-mindedly put Cathy and she never corrected me again.'

I thought of the efforts to which Catherine had gone in order to invest Steve with a citizen's proper status. Although the bank account and various other official documents that I found at the flat were mostly in the name of Catherine Morag Loudon, several semi-official letters and a lot of junk mail were addressed to Dr Steve Stevenz. I felt that had it been easy for her to do so, she would have changed her name to Steve on everything but I could have been wrong about that. She may have wanted to retain Cathy, too.

'Did you ever see her with other people?' I asked Karen. 'Did she ever have people to the flat?'

I was pretty sure what the answer would be, but I still harboured hopes of Catherine bringing home a friend, for tea and a smoke.

'Never,' Karen answered, decisively. 'If I saw her on the street she was by herself. But she went to the Methodist Centre and obviously there were lots of people there. The cafés, obviously there would have been other people there, too. I don't know if she knew people there or whether she'd just go in and have a cup of tea and be on her own but she went to places where there were other people.'

My tea was now chilly and grey. Staring into it, I considered how Catherine was always on the margins of everything, never at the centre. Although her illness put her firmly centre-stage many times she was only its agent. It was almost as if, when schizophrenia drew maximum attention to her and her actions, she herself was sidelined. There is a vessel-like quality about people within whom mental illness operates with such power and velocity that makes it easy to see why, historically, psychosis has been confused with diabolical possession.

So when I thought of Catherine alongside other people it brought less solace than it might have done. Catherine amidst a crowd could have been a pleasing thought but the image that it produced for me was only a little less isolating than one of her alone in her cold cell.

Karen was looking a little concerned.

'You know,' she said gently, 'I know of people who have a completely isolated life and don't like to go to places where there are other people. She wasn't like that.'

I sighed.

'She seemed to be out most of the day, pretty much every day,' Karen persisted, brightly. 'I'd pass her on the street or see her at all times of the day, as well as on the big main road that carries on from here up into other parts of Bristol. I live up there and quite often I'd see her at nine o'clock in the morning, up that way. It's a long way from here.'

I said, 'I got the impression from Steve Shepherd that she walked a lot.'

'I'm sure she did. I'd probably see her once every couple of weeks in the street. She would always stop and tell me a joke, and then wander off laughing.'

I could hear that laughter still. Disjointed laughter. Laughter, sometimes, fit to make you cry.

'What kind of jokes?' I asked.

'They were like cracker jokes,' Karen replied, 'if you know what I mean.'

I thought of the jokes in Catherine's letters. Knock knock, who's there?

'Yes, I know what you mean.'

'Silly jokes,' said Karen, 'but it always made me laugh that she saw me as someone that she wanted to tell a joke to. She'd tell me one and then wander off. Sometimes I'd get her to stand still for a second so I could say, "Are you okay?" and she'd say, "Yep!" and then off she'd go.'

'Yep!' How familiar was that rejoinder of Catherine's. How familiar, too, was Karen's description of Catherine's febrile quality. Jittery, that's the word our parents used to describe her inability to stand or sit still. But they used it also when she was manic and restless, swerving without warning between reason and madness, between conversations, rooms and countries, laughing and proselytising, her head full of persecution and strategy. Jittery. To my mind, it was a word of insufficient strength to support the weight of that which it described.

I imagined Catherine on the street outside her flat, Karen trying subtly to pin her down. I pictured her with her short hair, cigarette in hand.

'What did she used to wear?' I asked.

Unexpectedly, Karen laughed.

'I don't have to think about what she wore!' she exclaimed. 'She always wore trousers. Always had jeans or dark trousers on, and depending on the weather, she would either have a white shirt on or a shirt and jacket and sometimes a tie. Not always a tie but sometimes. The jacket, it was always dark. Apart from the shirt she wore sombre colours, blacks, greys, browns, greens, none of the clothing was ever brightly coloured. She was always very neat, very clean, very tidy. That's why we never had any concerns that she wasn't looking after herself. And her hair was always short and well cut, always in the same style, that never altered.'

I wondered why, in some of the self-portraits that I found in her flat, Catherine had long hair.

'That is strange,' said Karen. 'Did she have longer hair when she was young?'

'Only once,' I said. 'She went through a hippie phase when she wore it hanging down over her face. It was rather the opposite of her usual style.'

'I can't imagine her with long hair,' said Karen.

'And she was always smoking,' I said.

'Oh yes,' Karen agreed, wholeheartedly. 'She smoked.'

One of our relatives had laughed when I said I'd found Catherine's Rizla roll-ups. 'Good God,' she said, 'I used to roll them for her when we were teenagers. She must have been the only person in the world still rolling her own.'

I asked whether any of the other residents in the flats had had much contact with Catherine.

'I don't think they did,' Karen replied. 'But there was one thing: she did have quite a lot of different music that she would play and you could hear that sometimes. Quite often I had to sort that out.'

'What, because she played it too loudly?'

'Yeah. She would go through phases of playing the music very loudly, very late at night. I'd have to put a note through her door saying, "I don't know if you realise the time, and I appreciate that sometimes you don't but perhaps you could keep the volume down at night." And she would respond to that and everything would be fine.

'During the day she was out,' Karen continued, 'so she

didn't tend to play music then and therefore I didn't hear it, but I knew from the other tenants when she was playing music loudly at night because they told me. I always asked them, because I was interested, "What sort of music is it?" and they said, "Well, it's all sorts." Quite often it would be jazz, other times it would be classical, a lot of opera and piano music. I mean, some people here will just play something like drum and bass. Some people have the bass banging through the flats, which causes problems, but she wasn't doing that.

'Catherine was different,' Karen said. 'She played a lot of good music.' She sounded impressed, admiring even. 'It's just that she liked to play it loudly.'

I remembered Catherine's fear of sleeping in the dark, a fear that came home with her from India.

'I have a feeling,' I said, 'that she may have been more active at night. I have a hunch that that was when she did her paintings and writing.'

Karen nodded. 'That may well be why, yes.'

I said, 'I know this might sound weird to you but do you have any photographs of her at all?'

'No.'

'Steve told me that sometimes you have pictures of tenants.'

'Yeah, we take them if we have any social events,' said Karen.

I couldn't see Catherine attending anything that might be termed a 'social event'.

'Which she never attended,' Karen continued. 'I mean, they're open to everybody and we always put a note through the door or put a poster up, so she was well aware of them. And we'd take photos if we were doing a new leaflet or something but I hadn't any of her at all. I had the pictures that she did herself, up on the wall. She insisted that they went up. "Wouldn't it look nice here," she'd say. But that stopped after the first two or three years of knowing her. I wondered whether she felt safe enough with me that she didn't have to give me paintings any more to make sure I was there when she needed me.'

I imagined Catherine was simply giving the paintings to someone else by then. I didn't say as much, it would have been hurtful. But Catherine's attention span was short and many of her personal allegiances easily transferable. She probably did feel safe with Karen, but in the past, once she had established that someone was available to her she had a tendency to turn her attentions elsewhere. This wasn't always the case but it did seem to apply to people a bit like Karen, who featured in Catherine's life but were kept at its periphery.

'There's one thing I always remember,' Karen said, 'from a time when she was in Barrow.'

'Barrow?'

'Yeah, Barrow Gurney. That's the psychiatric hospital where she went when she was sectioned.'

Barrow Gurney. What a name.

'When she was in Barrow,' said Karen, 'one of the other tenants from this building happened to be there at the same time and he said that she played the piano. He said that she played it beautifully, that she played Beethoven sonatas. And I thought, I never knew that about her.'

I stared at Karen.

Beethoven sonatas. Those intense, vast, rambling pieces of music; heavy, sumptuous, full of chaos, beauty, passion and anger. The individual chords are so rich – in short, so full of notes – that they are fiendishly difficult to play. They require a wide stretch of the palm for a start, plus agility in the fingers, strength, power and deftness all at once.

'They're too big for my hands,' I used to complain to my piano teacher.

'Bloody nonsense,' he growled. 'Stop making excuses.'

But I never could play them well. I used to select the bits that were least tricky, and play those.

'Lovely,' said my teacher. 'Now let's hear the rest.'

Catherine could play the rest. It was she who could play the organ, after all.

And now, on an icy, wind-blasted railway platform, Karen had revealed my sister to me in a way I could never have anticipated: playing those lavish pieces years after she had, I believed, last touched a piano, her witness a man who knew them also. In my mind I saw them, these two people relegated, even by their own admission, to a psychiatric hospital with a name like death itself, sharing piano sonatas. That one of them had cared to relate the account of their performance was sufficient to floor me. Nothing I had already encountered could have prepared me for that knowledge. Stunned, I began to cry.

'Oh, sorry.' Karen was mortified. 'I didn't mean to upset you, I'm sorry.'

'It's okay.'

Karen leaned across the table to me.

'I just thought that it was a really lovely thing,' she explained, 'and something I didn't know. It just made me think that maybe she'd had a nice life or a happy childhood, because playing the piano is something that you work at and it also made her happy still. I mean, obviously there isn't a piano at the flats and I don't know if she ever played elsewhere.'

'Maybe there's one at the Methodist place,' I said, not hopefully.

'Maybe.' She shrugged, clearly embarrassed.

I found a tissue in my pocket and wiped my eyes.

'It's okay,' I reassured Karen. She was looking very worried.

'It's just a shock,' I said. 'I never realised.'

'I'm sorry,' she repeated. 'It just seemed like such a lovely thing.'

In Retreat

Returning home on the train, I gave up on my book and picked up a newspaper left on the seat beside me. Pleased, because it was an unspeakably lousy one of a kind I like secretly to read, I learned that Farrah Fawcett, one-time TV star and Seventies icon, denied going on the US's David Letterman show 'in an altered state', by which I assumed she meant alcohol or some other drug. And I wondered then, as I looked out of the window at the Wiltshire villages speeding by: What is an 'unaltered' state? Leaving aside treatments for illness, or the use of mind- or mood-affecting substances, there is no actual alternative to anyone in his or her natural state. There is no parallel universe known to us, where better, happier versions of ourselves exist.

When Catherine was in her mid-thirties and already in retreat from whatever it was that pained her about her own femininity, I was in my early twenties and on a happy adventure with all that pleased me about mine. I've often wondered whether this alone makes her and me so radically different that our kinship might as well be regarded as mere genetic detail, a blip of DNA and circumstance, and little more. We ate the same food at the same table, cooked by the same mother, in the shelter of whose love we both grew. The photographs of a tiny Catherine on our father's lap are as good as identical to photographs of the rest of us in similar childhood embraces. So the soil was no different. It wasn't as if Catherine fell on unaccountably stony ground.

Yet she might as well have done, for while the rest of us prospered she faltered. She failed to appreciate, or so I have been told, the fundamental difference between right and wrong, good and bad, even love and indifference. In a rudimentary sense, the rest of us understood these things by early childhood. Most children do. But Catherine, our mother says, seemed as close to amoral as it is possible to be, remaining curiously unmoved by petty wrongdoing and unperturbed by her deceits against others. And while the rest of us obviously did not react the same way to different things, our reactions, according to our mother, fell within the same category of response. Catherine's response was almost always different from everyone else's and it was never predictable. When it was, it was a surprise.

For a time, there was a disorderly clump of wheat that grew in our parents' garden, just where the lawn met the orchard. It was the legacy of Catherine's relationship with the cockerel known as Cocky whom she was deputed to feed in the mornings, along with the other hens and bantams that we kept at the time. Cocky was an outright thug, with a tendency to random attacks. Catherine was too frightened to go near him so she stayed close to the house instead, tipping the wheat-grain into the flowerbed at the edge of the lawn and returning to the sanctuary of the kitchen with her secret of the un-fed birds. Ultimately, she was discovered and relieved of all duties pertaining to hens. In the meantime, Cocky and his ilk never starved, though some came to perilous ends via foxes and dogs. One, who preferred to roost in long grass rather than the low branches customarily favoured by bantams, was accidentally chewed up by a lawn-mower.

I don't blame Catherine for wanting to avoid that mean old bird. I was attacked by Cocky when I was small. He came at me from behind, which meant I was pecked in the backs of the knees rather than the face (small comfort at the time), and I, too, would not go near him. But because the things that routinely worried or scared other people engendered in Catherine not so much a lack of fear as a basic disregard, it was a surprise when her responses matched those of other people. It was a shock when she seemed briefly to occupy the same emotional and psychological spaces as the rest of us. Normal behaviour from her was unexpected because it was almost impossible to anticipate. For me, that clump of wheat represented Catherine's sanity.

Most of the time, however, Catherine's relationship with the world around her was governed by her illness. When she was having severe schizophrenic episodes it was impossible for anyone to predict what she might do next. It was also impossible for Catherine to rely on the information that she received from outside because whatever was going on in her brain corrupted it. Paranoia would take over and delusions dominate. Beleaguered by the voices in her head the saner Catherine, with her wit and her curious, spiky charm, would be overwhelmed by an awful egocentricity.

Because her illness functioned like a poisoned filter, Catherine's interior world was driven by the fearsome unpredictability of her exterior one. Harmless words or gestures were perceived as threats. People who were not there, or did not exist, were believed to be present. The voices that only she could hear issued mandates to behave wilfully or dangerously. While it was certainly hard for other people to cope with Catherine when she was crazy, it was probably harder still for Catherine to cope with herself. It is not surprising that she became alarmed and suspicious. It is logical that she came to guard her privacy so ferociously.

My husband used to work with a New York PR man called John Scanlon. Scanlon (as he was known to all) was vast of girth and character, and in a culture of he-who-works-longest-wins he was pretty refreshing. Damned if he was going to get through the day without a good snooze, he liked to sleep after lunch on the billowing cushions of his Manhattan office sofa, come hell or high water. If you phoned him during his siesta you would speak instead to his colleague, Peter Hirsch, who would say to you, deep irony disguised by perfect American manners, 'I'm sorry, but John Scanlon is currently disavailable.'

I like 'disavailable'. I like the idea of being neither available nor unavailable. It sounds both more absolute and more slippery. Just as Scanlon was 'disavailable', I came to think of Catherine as 'disinvolved', which suggests something altogether less overt than uninvolved. Uninvolved implies an active decision not to partake. Disinvolved (would there were such a word) suggests a lack of involvement which the person to whom it refers is probably not even aware of.

That doesn't mean that a lack of participation is not difficult or painful for the disinvolved. Without actually wishing for anything specific, a person can still realise that things might be easier if they were different. I know that Catherine was always aware of her status as an outsider. I know, because I have been told, that she felt unlike other children and was occasionally reduced to tears by her sense of not belonging. I think this sense of hers was profound. She didn't feel like other girls. She didn't dress like them, look like them or react like them. She believed she was made differently. She made it clear on more than one occasion that she felt biologically wrong. Maybe she was. Maybe Steve was a more reasonable, inevitable outcome for her than anyone could have known. Maybe in addition to the schizophrenia she was lumbered with there was something else to deal with, too, a chromosomal abnormality perhaps, or a hormonal one. Nobody knows.

It is fruitless to speculate upon an alternative version of Catherine, a Catherine free of schizophrenia, for schizophrenic is not just what she was, it's who she was. Whatever its causes, the illness was a component part of her fabric, its effects deeply emblazoned on every portion of her being. The healthy version of Catherine – the different kind of artist she might have been, the musician and wit, the keeper of dogs and a quiet home – exists only in a wistful imagination.

People often describe the mentally ill as 'not themselves' and 'not all there', and when they do, I wonder if they realise what they are saying. I wonder if they mean to imply that people like my sister are missing something. If they are, then they are implying also that the mentally ill exist only partially. That notion might be quite comforting for those who find it hard to accept that the strangers in our midst are as whole as the rest of us, but it rests upon a stunning misconception. The mentally ill are not like ill-manufactured jigsaw puzzles. They are like the rest of us, unique and complex organisms, subject to change in the making.

So while in some individual cases there might be a mutated gene here, or a reduced neurotransmitter there, these things are not missing in the sense that they can be located elsewhere. And even those people with mental illnesses attributable to a lack of something specific are most definitely 'all there', for they are all there is. After all, some of us lack humour, humility or sensitivity but this is not regarded as a fundamental problem, even though deficiency of these characteristics can prove disabling in many areas of life.

A friend of mine nursed his wife for many years before her death as she declined steadily into premature senility. She had Alzheimer's disease. When I first met them, the illness had already set right in to her. Elisabeth would wander around their house serene but fairly oblivious to the activities around her and to furniture that stood in her way. She needed help dressing and eating. She needed guiding to a table otherwise she blundered.

'The worst part,' said Hugh, 'is not this. It was when the illness started. I found her on the bed one day, crying. It was just before she was diagnosed. She said, "I know what's happening to me, I know what's happening. I'm losing my mind." It was awful.'

I never had a conversation with Elisabeth, though she had once been a keen conversationalist. It wasn't possible. She muttered short phrases to herself, repeating them over and over again. She was friendly to others, meaning that she was calm in their presence and interested in looking at them, but she had no idea who I was or who most people were. She was definitely aware that Hugh was important to her and was loving towards him but that was about as far as her ability to relate to someone else went.

Elisabeth had done what so many women did and still do. She had raised three children, run a home, looked after her husband while he worked long hours, long weeks, long years. She had supported her family and like most women of her generation had put any desires beyond it a long way down the list. She was a woman of intellectual capability and culinary talent, someone who talked, read and cooked wonderful food. When I met her, she was a shell.

For a long time I was haunted by Elisabeth, vexed partly by the question of where she – the Elisabeth of the past whom I had never met – had gone, but also by the thought that she might not have gone at all. Nobody knows where the dead go, if indeed they go anywhere at all, but the living? Here was someone still alive and seemingly empty, or near enough, with the better part of her faculties drained from her. But what if she was not empty? What if, still present inside this woman, was the wife who knew what was happening to her, the mother who cooked a thousand Sunday lunches? What if, when I was introduced to Elisabeth each time I visited her house, she knew perfectly well who I was, had heard it all before, but simply could not communicate thus? Was there, inside the mind we all assumed she had lost, a lost person instead, with things that she wanted to say but could not find the words for, feelings she wished to share but could no longer describe?

It's a nightmarish thought. It's also a futile thought for the overwhelming odds are that Elisabeth's oblivion was just that. The chances are that she was spared – ultimately at least – from the indignities and vicissitudes of her own decline, separated from the appalling fear of her impending degeneration by the degeneration itself. The French have a phrase, *bien dans sa peau*, meaning that someone is comfortable within their own skin. Elisabeth seemed perfectly comfortable in her own skin when I knew her, probably because the mechanism for experiencing and understanding loss was all but destroyed. Put another way, I don't think she had a clue what had happened to her. She didn't know to mourn her own disappearance.

For some it is not so. For some, being locked inside is something they are aware of. I believe that Catherine felt incarcerated in her own skin and if she was as bedevilled by her mind as it appears then her attempt to distance herself from the body which contained it seems entirely natural. She believed she had been tortured in a Tibetan jail. I believe she was tortured in her own.

Nevertheless, I want to believe that Catherine chose. I want to think that her illness didn't make her a total prisoner, even unto her own thoughts. But I am not at all sure. I like to imagine that she chose a home for her soul in Steve. I like to think she did it in much the same way that a transvestite might choose to adopt an alter ego on occasions, whilst maintaining the name and persona by which he is known for the rest of the time. But I suspect that those are fond imaginings. I don't really believe that transvestites choose to cross-dress because I have always been under the impression that the act of cross-dressing is driven more by imperative than choice, by need rather than desire. And thus I don't believe that Catherine chose Steve, not really.

But still I don't know where Steve came from and I think it's a fair bet that Catherine didn't know, either. I want to suppose that Catherine created him but that is only conjecture. I don't even know why Steve was Steve and not, say, Dave, Phil or Matt. I do know that Catherine was drawn to the poet Stevie Smith when she was younger but to make a connection between that and her later persona seems a bit arbitrary. Perhaps Steve just evolved over time. Maybe he was more of an accident than a design. It is possible that Catherine fell into a relationship with him in the way that people often fall into relationships with one another, by degrees and without plans.

Certainly, Steve as a creation begs several questions, especially when you consider the exterior chaos of an internal life so brutally compromised by an illness that works from the inside out. He could be understood in several ways. He could be viewed as a form of welcome relief for Catherine from the burden of her self. He could be seen as the burden and not the respite. He could be perceived as a benign manifestation of some much less benign demons, as a residue of chaos but not intrinsically disordered. Personally, however, I find it difficult to think of him as anything less than the manifestation of a mighty compulsion of Catherine's to flee from something terrifying.

The imagination can provide emancipation and deliverance when life cannot. But what happens when the mind is the place from which someone needs deliverance? Catherine heard voices, she lived in perpetual fear of persecution. Some schizophrenics have visual hallucinations, they see people or objects and believe instead that they are standing before strange and terrifying beasts. It's little wonder that some of them commit suicide.

So Catherine's taking of residency in Steve may well have been an imaginative choice that improved the quality of her life. But what if it wasn't as simple as that? Even if Steve was the result of choice on Catherine's part, choice itself can be motivated by different things. Choice is not always the product of will or desire. Choice is sometimes no more than an escape bid, which means that the place where someone ends up is wrongly regarded as his or her favoured destination. In Catherine's case, Steve was where she ended up. That does not mean he was where she really wished to be.

This is why I doubt that Catherine's freedom from the most basic aspects of her identity – her name, her sex – was motivated primarily by a sense of possible alternatives. I believe instead that her liberation from the self she found it so painful to inhabit was entirely regulated by her illness. Steve may have provided a safe haven for her but I can't believe that he provided true liberty, by which I suppose I mean contentment, *bien dans sa peau*. I am certain he improved things for Catherine and I'd love to think that he stood for everything Catherine felt that she was, or wished to be. But I have reservations about him. For me, Steve has come to represent instead some fundamental things – a man, first and foremost – that Catherine was not. I want to regard him as a great liberator. I fear he may instead have been a new and different form of encumbrance.

A friend of mine changed her Christian name by deed poll when she was eighteen. She says the rejection implicit in the decision was in no way profound, that it was a simple matter of ditching a name she didn't like in favour of one that she did. Privately, I'm generally inclined to believe that decisions of this kind are psychologically loaded in some way but that's what she says and I believe her. And why shouldn't I? What do I know about these things?

Nothing, is the answer.

I know nothing at all about these things.

Stevie

The morning I met Richard McKay, I was exhausted. It seemed suddenly rather hopeless, the way I had cast myself into a world full of strangers. It felt so foreign, this journey of mine into my sister's past; so foreign and so bleak.

He welcomed me into the large Victorian presbytery in which he lived, a kindly Roman Catholic priest alone in a sparsely-furnished, vast-roomed house. In the kitchen, he made tea and gentle chat. He assured me that the next two hours were all mine. He put on his answer-phone and in the sitting room he shut the door so I was cocooned from other people in the house and everything else outside it. Even with the muffled background whirr of passing cars it was like sitting in the hush of a public library.

I thought of the invocation, *Come to me, ye weary, and I will give ye rest*. It had meaning for me that morning.

'You knew my sister as Stevie,' I said, as we settled into armchairs. I hadn't the energy for the gentle easing of myself into my sister's life that day.

When Richard spoke, his voice was even.

'Yes, that's right.'

'How long did you know her for?'

'Well,' said Richard, putting his hands together and making a steeple shape under his chin with his two forefingers, 'I met her soon after I came here, and I came here five years ago now.'

'Did she come to services at the church?'

'Occasionally,' said Richard. 'She would tend to come into a service and then go round to the Lady Chapel, or one of the other chapels. She would walk around during the service and then walk out again.'

I could see Catherine pacing our parents' house and garden; not up and down like a caged animal but erratically, restlessly.

'She found it difficult to stay still,' said Richard, confirming what I already knew, 'but she was there and I think that was important to her. She often wanted to light candles, so she'd go into the Lady Chapel because we have little candle stands there, and she'd light a few candles and kneel or sit and pray. That was not unusual for her.'

I lit a candle for you today, she wrote to me in one of her letters. Probably she did so in Richard's church.

He said, 'I noticed in the last eighteen months seeing less and less of her; less of her around in the area and certainly less of her coming into the church. But for the first couple of years I was here she was a not infrequent visitor.'

I told him that for the last eighteen months of her life she was seriously ill.

'Right,' he said, gently.

Richard had an immensely sympathetic air. There was also something quite tough about him although he lacked obvious ego. If Catherine chose to spend time with him, then she chose well.

'Did she talk to you much?' I asked.

'She did sometimes, yes. In the first couple of years, she certainly did. Sometimes she was really quite lucid, other times she would get very angry, irrationally angry for no reason. She'd shout at you. But you knew it was an illness, so you really didn't mind.'

I thought of the people you see in the street sometimes, people who are obviously sick, hurling abuse to left and right. My sister, was she one of them, some of the time?

'Was it personal abuse she shouted at you?'

'Yeah, I suppose so,' said Richard mildly, 'a bit.'

I wondered, amazed, what she could have found to abuse in Richard.

'Like what? Did she swear at you?'

'Oh yeah,' he said. 'But compared with the swearing you have round here it wasn't too bad. On the Richter Scale, it was fairly low.'

I said, 'You say she got irrationally angry.'

'Yes.'

'Was her anger irrational inasmuch as you didn't understand why she was angry,' I asked, 'or was it irrational because she was angry about something that it didn't make sense to be angry about?'

Richard considered the question.

'Well, it could be either,' he said, in measured tones. 'She would walk into the church and shout, and occasionally she did it in the middle of a service. She would say what hypocrites we were, and nothing provoked it, put it that way; so it was irrational in the sense that it didn't seem triggered by anything that we had done.'

'How did you react?'

'Oh, we'd just ignore it. Just let it happen. Don't worry about it.'

'You didn't try and remove her?'

Richard stared at me. He didn't look shocked but he did look as if something like that would never have occurred to him.

'Oh no,' he said. 'No, no, no. As you will know, if you're a parish in the inner city you become very tolerant of things. You have drunks coming in to church and shouting sometimes, and obviously if it becomes intolerably disruptive that's another matter. But somebody coming in, shouting, and then going out again, you just let that ride; and I think quite a lot of people knew Stevie and made allowances.'

Allowances. What a beautiful word it was all of a sudden; how capacious the tolerance and understanding it both described and accommodated.

'When she was angry or distressed,' I said, 'did she mention specific things that you can remember, specific events, or places, or people?'

He thought.

'No,' he replied.

'Not Tibet?'

Richard shook his head.

'Funny you mention Tibet,' he said. 'I was following a car today that had a *Free Tibet* sticker on, and I was thinking about that situation. But no, she didn't mention it. I know that she was very committed to Amnesty International because I used to pay her membership for her.'

'That was nice of you.'

Richard made a self-effacing gesture with his hands.

'Well, I found it really interesting that she wanted me to do that. Though she never asked for money,' he added, quite emphatically. 'I've loads and loads of people ask me on the door for money. She never did. The only thing she ever asked me to pay for was her membership of Amnesty International, and she'd occasionally come and talk to me about it for a few minutes. But all our conversations were brief ones because she never seemed to want more than a five-minute conversation.'

I smiled at him and said, 'That seems to have been the norm.'

'Yes,' he replied.

He screwed up his face into a frown.

'I wish I could remember them better but they didn't hang together well. Sometimes they made no sense. Sometimes they were statements rather than conversations. She'd come and say something and then go away again. With me, for understandable reasons, quite often it was to do with religion.'

'Do you remember what she said about it?'

'No, I can't. But I remember she would make these staccato statements from time to time.'

'About God?'

'Yes. Sometimes, when she was angry.'

'Was she angry with God?'

Richard paused for a moment.

'Don't think so. I think she was angry with people, with hypocrisy, mostly.'

'Catherine always had difficulty with hypocrisy.'

I used to admire her for it, her intense dislike of those who failed to practise what they preached, although it didn't stop her behaving very badly towards the family sometimes. It didn't stop her taking advantage whilst angrily reminding anyone who countered her that she was on a path to enlightenment and therefore her mind was on higher things than being nice to people.

I wasn't sure what Richard knew about Catherine's religious background.

'Did you know she became a Roman Catholic?' I asked him.

He thought for a moment.

'Did I know that? I'm not sure she ever told me. I had this feeling she might have been a Catholic.'

'Well, she is . . . was. She became one. We're not a Catholic family.'

'It makes sense to me,' said Richard, thoughtfully. 'It definitely makes sense to me.'

I wondered what he meant by that. I suppose he meant he could detect a newly-minted Catholic from one born into the culture and religion. Everyone has an instinctive feel for someone not of their tribe.

'She was pretty active for a while,' I said. 'She went to church every day but I know from what she told us that she stopped after a couple of years. Do you know if she was coming to this particular church before you came here?'

'I think she was,' Richard replied, 'because people knew her when I arrived here.'

'Was there anybody in the congregation she knew well or talked to regularly?'

'I'm not sure there was but the person who might know best is somebody called Betty Wear.'

'She's in the congregation here?'

'Yes.'

I said, 'I know that she went to see a nun because Steve Shepherd, who's the caretaker at the flats, told me. But I haven't found her yet. It was a Sister Margaret, Steve thought.'

'Sister Margaret.' Richard frowned, then nodded slowly. 'In that case, I think she's most likely to have been from one of two nearby Communities.'

I thought of all those phone calls.

'Yes,' I said. 'I narrowed it down to one myself. I'm still waiting to hear from the Sisters of Saint Joseph.'

'They'd be a good bet,' he said, enthusiastically. 'I was going to suggest that you phoned them. And they have a lot of contact with this church.'

'Well, that's helpful, thank you. Do you think Betty Wear would mind if I got in touch with her?'

'No, she wouldn't mind at all. She certainly knew Stevie.'

Stevie. It still sounded odd to me.

'I never knew her as anything else,' Richard added, slightly apologetically. 'Steve or Stevie.'

I recalled my phone conversation with George, the owner of the grocery shop next to Richard's church. He had referred to Catherine as Cathy, or Cath. There was no mention from him of Stevie.

I said to Richard, 'You said to me when we spoke on the phone that she got angry if she was referred to as a woman.'

He nodded.

'I was thinking about this coming here,' he said, 'I was thinking about Stevie. I had to say Mass on the other side of the city and I got held up in a traffic jam and was afraid I was going to be late for you, and I remembered having to write a letter for her, I don't know quite why.'

'For Amnesty, perhaps?' I suggested.

'No, it wasn't Amnesty. I think it was something to do with housing. But I remember writing a letter for her and describing her as "she", and she got very angry. "I'm not a woman!" she said. "People say that about me but I'm not!" She got really angry.'

Richard laughed.

He added, 'So I found another way of expressing what I needed to that didn't present the problem.'

When I was still a teenager, my friends used to ask me what this mysterious sister of mine looked like. I gave no proper answer, ever. I was embarrassed by Catherine's lack of femininity, ashamed even. I worried that somehow her mannishness might reflect poorly upon the high glamour of my mini-skirts and frosted pink lipstick. Aged fifteen and sixteen, I wanted prettiness not just for myself but by association. Older, I was more candid. 'You wouldn't know whether she was a man or woman,' I'd say, 'at least, not from just looking at her.'

I said, 'It seems that she looked the same now as she used to years ago. She didn't look very feminine then.'

'No,' Richard agreed, 'she never looked feminine but you could tell she was a woman, even though she was clearly trying to make herself look like a man. And I think she was reasonably successful in that because you'd still have a doubt in your mind. You'd think, "She's a woman . . . Or is she?" So when she protested that time, it made me think perhaps I'd got it wrong after all.'

I thought how we tend to believe what we're told, even when our instincts tell us something else.

'But her voice must have been a giveaway,' I said. 'Surely.'

If I concentrate, I can still hear Catherine's voice. It was high-pitched, thin, and a little dry from all the smoking. It certainly contained no baritone, nor even much contralto.

'Well, it was a higher range than would be normal for a man,' Richard agreed, 'but there are some men who have very high-pitched voices so she could carry it off reasonably well.'

I said, 'This might sound like a stupid question but when you saw her walking around the place, was her bearing that of someone who was closed in or looking outwards? Do you remember?'

Richard smiled.

'Yes, I do. She had a slightly loping walk, and if I can put it this way,' he said, very politely, 'which is not the politically correct way of putting it, you knew she wasn't well and there was a problem. You could tell she was a little odd just by the way she walked; because some people you can tell by their walk, can't you.'

'You can.'

'It was that rather staccato walk that I've seen in other people who are not well. She was sometimes a bit bowed but usually very erect.'

I explained that in my mind's eye she had always been bowed, brought low by the travails of a life lived within the confines of her illness.

'Oh no,' said Richard. 'No, you got the impression of actually quite a strong person, maybe mentally vulnerable but a real survivor.'

'So what was she like towards you when she wasn't hostile?'

'Very friendly,' he answered. 'She would talk a lot when in good humour. She would talk to herself at times as well. Sometimes she'd be laughing to herself.'

Always she'd be laughing to herself, it seemed to me, all those years ago, giggling conspiratorially as she rolled another cigarette.

'I had two dogs at one stage,' said Richard, brightly, 'my own dog and then when my parents came to live with me, we had my parents' dog. And I remember Stevie used to like stroking the dogs. She would sit a lot just outside the grocers' shop, leaning against the wall on her haunches, and if I was passing by with the dogs she would sometimes pet them.' He added, chuckling, 'She would sometimes address the dogs rather than me but that's not unusual.'

I remembered Catherine at home with her much-loved dog, Jenny. Jenny was the only dog in family memory who could do tricks and walk to heel without a lead, or sit and wait obediently outside a shop, because Catherine was the only person in the family with the patience to train a dog as well as that. She had a gift with dogs.

'Hers was the best trained dog in the family,' I remarked. 'Jenny. She adored her.'

There was a silence, which neither of us sought to fill. Perhaps Richard was thinking of Catherine and his dogs. I was. I could see her rubbing their backs and nuzzling the loose folds of skin around their jaws. I could see her with Jenny on the lawn at home.

'It's funny, isn't it,' I said, finally, 'how she could be Stevie with you but Cathy at the shop. You're within a stone's throw of the shop.'

'That is interesting,' Richard agreed.

'And it seems that the same was true at the general practice,' I said. 'Apparently she insisted on being known as

Stevie to the practice nurse, but to her GP she was Cathy.'

'That's actually quite sophisticated.' Richard was impressed. 'Being able to be one thing to this person, and one thing to another.'

And being able to be two things to yourself, I thought. Being Cathy inside a shop and Stevie on the pavement outside, that's sophisticated. That's something beyond the parameters of most people's experiences. I wondered what went on inside my sister's head when she ran into Richard within inches of George. Was there any conflict therein?

'But it doesn't surprise me,' Richard remarked. 'It was quite clear that here was a very intelligent person who obviously had quite a severe condition.'

I thought of the many and vivid words that people who came across my sister might have used to describe her. I imagine very few of them would have said, 'She's a schizophrenic, most likely.'

'Did you have any hunch what her condition was?' I asked.

'Yes,' said Richard. 'Oh yes.'

He had probably known a few like Catherine.

'You're right that she was intelligent,' I said. 'She was. And do you know, I found something interesting when I looked at some of her notebooks. A lot of what's in them doesn't make sense, and is disturbing, but it was clear that she was either self-studying medicine or believed she was a doctor. She had called herself not just Stevie but Dr Steven Stevenz.'

Richard raised an eyebrow.

'The notebooks containing her medical studies,' I continued, 'they were lucid and technically accurate. I imagine a lot of what was in them had been copied from textbooks. But what interested me were the areas that interested her. There was no reference to schizophrenia or cancer, both of which she had.

She was fascinated by blood diseases: sickle-cell anaemia, hepatitis, HIV. And I don't know where her interest in those things came from.'

'No,' said Richard, 'but then I would describe her as one of the "street people". Although she obviously had her own flat, she tended to live on the street more than anywhere else and HIV, AIDS, hepatitis, they're common currency of conversation on the street because so many on the street are HIV-positive.'

'I see.'

'So it might be that she was interested because that was part of the world that she was sharing in.'

'Perhaps on the street she found a community where she could be herself without it being a problem, or too much remarked upon,' I suggested.

Richard nodded vigorously.

'Yes,' he said. 'I think that's absolutely right.'

I remembered that in the course of trying to track down the nun who knew Catherine, I phoned a voluntary organisation for the homeless in Bristol, run by a group of Roman Catholics called the Cyrenians. I knew Catherine had been there because she had told us about it, in letters home. On the end of the phone was a woman called Sonya who had known Catherine for a short while.

'She used to do these crazy things,' said Sonya. 'We'd have people turn up here at the centre, and if they were homeless and it was their first day in Bristol, or their first night out of prison, Catherine would say, "Oh, you can come and kip at my place." '

'That's nice,' I said, rather proudly, while considering without much surprise the flexibility of the closed-door policy that Catherine had applied to us.

'Well, yes,' said Sonya, doubtfully, 'but I was very worried by it. I mean, she could have been murdered!'

She said it with some relish.

'Well, she wasn't,' I replied.

'No,' said Sonya, 'luckily.'

I said to Richard, 'I think the fact that her friends were people who had serious difficulties is quite significant.'

'There are very strong bonds between street people,' he said. 'In a way that's giving them a label, and I don't like giving labels, but nonetheless they do have strong bonds. They have their own way of relating to each other which isn't perhaps what we would recognise as good relationships, because there can be quite a lot of aggression and falling in and out. There's a mixture of loyalty and disloyalty and both seem to co-exist quite easily, so while it can be a chaotic lifestyle, it does mean that on the street you're accepted for what you present yourself to be without any questions asked and without anybody being disturbed by it. That's a very positive value. The rest of us seem to require people to fit into some kind of mould.'

That doesn't apply to my family, I thought; not to my generous, liberal parents. But then I considered the things that Catherine had been raised to do. I thought about the house she had grown up in and her expensive education. I thought about her speaking French and painting, particular skills that were regarded, a century before, as basics for a cultivated woman. I thought about the various conditional offers from universities to read Art, abandoned because school expulsion and drug-taking did not fall within those conditions. I recalled Catherine's ability to distinguish Corelli from Vivaldi, while preferring Bob Dylan.

Catherine never put two fingers up at her education but it's quite possible that she found the possibilities it represented oppressive. She was never required by anyone to do anything in particular and yet it is hard to disentangle opportunity from expectation. You are not given piano lessons unless playing the piano is regarded as valuable in some way. You are not encouraged to speak foreign languages unless it is supposed that one day you may need them. You are not filled with these good things in the expectation that you will end up behind a locked door, though no loving parent would deny them to you even if they knew that your outcome was likely to be less than happy. But if you do end up behind a locked door, do you perhaps, when considering the many doors open to you in the past, feel resentful or angry? Do you imagine yourself a disappointment? Is that part of the reason that you cannot face the people who love you for who you are, because you believe – however mistakenly – that they see you only for what you are not?

As a parent, you offer all you can to your children without condition, especially your love. I know our parents did. But proximity alone can produce pressures of its own. I don't for one second believe that Catherine's illness had as its underlying cause a background replete with choice and expectation, because a background with none would have presented different challenges to a vulnerable child. Catherine did not find family life easy but I don't think she would have found any family life easy. Most schizophrenics do not. But a schizophrenic child or teenager can look, to those with no understanding of the illness, simply like the family rebel, and therefore the family is mistakenly held to account for behaviours and outcomes that probably have their origins quite elsewhere.

I said, 'Catherine's care worker told me something strange.'

I recounted the story of the Beethoven sonatas, a story, it occurred to me suddenly, that was now third-hand.

'Goodness,' he said.

'Do you have a piano in your church?'

'We don't have a piano. We do have an organ but she never asked to play it.'

I sighed.

I said, 'I guess she was just able to sit down and play after all those years.'

It was perfectly possible. I've barely touched my piano for a decade but there are still things I can play, badly.

I added, 'Once something's really in your fingers, it tends to stay there.'

Richard sat up straighter all of a sudden.

'Can I just say,' he interjected, 'because I've just remembered it, she always wore this particular bag. She was always carrying a bag over her shoulder.'

'What sort of bag?'

'It was a briefcase-type bag, squarish.'

'When you say briefcase-type, was it hard?'

'No, soft.'

'I think I might have it. Was it brown leather?'

'Might have been. I think so. It was over her back usually, sometimes over her front. It was a very distinctive look, that and her anorak. And short, short, cropped hair, she had very short hair.'

Catherine's hair. It looked as if it had been a month out of the Army. As a child, I wished that she would grow it, believing that with long hair she would be physically transformed into a soft-focus, fairy-tale sister. When once she did allow it to grow, it fell about her face, extinguishing her features.

'Did she ever mention family to you?' I asked.

'No.'

'Right. And I'm quite sure you didn't ask her questions.'

'No,' said Richard, 'and she certainly gave off vibes that you shouldn't. If you tried to probe at all, the shutters would go down and she would flare up at you.'

'She was good at vibes,' I said. 'I even felt them in her flat.'

'I'm not surprised.'

I said, 'I'm sure she was there when I went in with my husband. But I'm also pretty sure she understood why I was there. I don't know why I feel that,' I added, wondering as I had before whether it was pure self-justification, 'but I do.'

Richard nodded.

'I told you about going to see her in hospital in the mortuary, didn't I?'

'You did.'

'That was quite an extraordinary experience. So calm. I could have sat there all day just to absorb the calm because it had a quality unlike any other calm I've ever known.'

'I understand,' said Richard, and he sounded as if he did. 'It's a strange presence-absence, isn't it.'

'Yes,' I said, 'that's exactly what it was like.'

'It's like, this isn't the same person and yet there is something of them here, very strongly.'

'Yes,' I said. 'Yes. And the peace of it was just extraordinary, because I felt she was at peace, I really did.'

'Oh yes,' said Richard. 'I have no problem believing that at all.'

I smiled at him, a man with no problem believing.

'Well, I wouldn't expect you to,' I said, 'assuming that your faith is pretty intact.'

'Sure,' he replied, smiling too, 'but also, from my many experiences with death, I believe that very often the powerful experiences come from people like Stevie. When somebody's had a very disturbed life there can be enormous peace.'

He paused.

'I'm quite involved in the healing ministry', he said, and the way he said 'quite involved' suggested that the term was an understatement, 'and I often say that death is the ultimate healing. You can feel it at funerals sometimes.'

'Really?'

'Yes.'

I said, 'I found myself most strongly hoping for a life after death when Catherine died, for some sort of mysterious continuation.'

He nodded.

'I mean, I would so love to see her again. And it's not the wanting to see someone that's borne of grief, it's just the sense that it would be really lovely to see her whole, you know.'

'I do,' said Richard. 'I do.'

'Immediately after she died, I was very frightened that she would appear to me unexpectedly. Now, I rather wish she would.'

'I can understand that,' said Richard.

I felt relieved.

'I think your feelings are important,' he said, simply, 'because you have sensed the healing in Stevie, you've felt it. It's why, when I preach at funerals, I say that death is the ultimate healing because it's in death that we finally become who we are.'

'I hope so,' I said. 'I really do.'

Around and Around

Up and down and around and around I went.

To Bristol it would say in my diary. And I'd get on the train, or into the car, and make my way just a little bit further into Catherine's life.

It wasn't all as straightforward as the meetings with Karen and Richard.

I spent a long time on the phone. I spoke to some people who had known my sister and to an awful lot that had not.

Once, I drove all the way to Bristol only to find that the person who had arranged to meet me at her workplace was at home, unwell. She hadn't thought to let me know. I sat in my car and cried, furious at the wasted time and energy of it all, before turning around to drive the 80 miles home again. Attempting to make another appointment with her proved fruitless.

I went twice to the Midland Road Methodist Centre where I'd been told, by Karen, that Catherine used to go for lunch. But it was shut both times. I copied down the telephone number that was on a piece of paper stuck to the window in the door.

I rang a few times, and finally I got hold of a volunteer called Nicola.

'Yeah, I knew Cathy,' she said. 'She came to the Centre quite a lot.'

Nicola also used to see Catherine walking around the city, or foraging in skips.

'She made picture frames with materials she got from them,' Nicola explained. 'She was very resourceful and very selective with her materials. She wouldn't work with just anything. She was very selective about people, too. I think she had a few people she could trust, and she talked just to them.'

Everyone I spoke to had been struck by Catherine's appearance.

'She loved clothes,' said Nicola, 'especially men's ties, and jewellery. She had lovely jewellery. I remember one particular ring, it had a Mona Lisa on it. I think there was a part of her that was very female. She was very sensitive, and really into art and music, especially jazz.'

Nicola asked me about Catherine's funeral. There was some regret in her voice. I explained that at that stage we hadn't known whom, in Bristol, to invite.

'Well, I would've come to her funeral, definitely,' she said, 'if I'd known about it.'

From the nurses at the Bristol Royal Infirmary I had learned that Catherine was looked after by a hospital social worker whose name was Carol. It was the job of the hospital social worker to make it possible for Catherine to die comfortably at home, which confused me, because Catherine didn't die at home, she died in hospital.

I managed to get hold of Carol on the phone.

'I take people as I find them,' said Carol, 'and your sister was always friendly and polite to me, she was no trouble. She had a good sense of humour. She didn't want the mobile phone I gave her, so she made quite a lot of jokes about that, but that was about the only time she objected to anything; although she took it in the end.'

I thought about the classic schizophrenics' fear of things like televisions, radios and telephones. I thought how many of them believe, as Catherine had, that they are devices used by the Secret Services to spy on or manipulate them. Did Carol have any idea what she was doing when she pressed that mobile phone upon my sister?

I said I was confused by the fact that there were arrangements for Catherine to return to her flat to die.

'That wasn't me,' said Carol. 'That was Louise.'

She didn't really want to see me, this Louise. It was obvious, the moment I arrived. I think she felt compromised by my request to talk to her, and she hadn't managed to say no quickly enough on the phone. She was probably kicking herself.

She said to me straight away, 'You look similar. I can see the family resemblance,' and she gestured towards a large committee room across the corridor from her office, which was on the fourth floor of a building in the centre of the city.

'We can go in here,' she said.

We sat on hard, orange plastic chairs. She didn't offer me a cup of tea and she didn't want to talk. She didn't say so. She didn't need to. Her arms were folded tightly across her chest.

I wasn't really surprised. She was a social worker, after all, and they get lots of flak, all the time. Perhaps she thought I was going to give her flak. Perhaps she had seen Catherine as a victim and she saw me now as something of an oppressor, as a negligent relative who only now, after Catherine's death, was showing any kind of interest in her.

However she regarded me, she saw Catherine as Stevie, and Stevie as feminine. Yet another variation.

She said that Stevie was very keen to leave hospital and die at home. She made it clear that she and her colleagues had done everything they could to make that possible. This was because, according to Louise, Stevie had said she didn't want to go into a hospice, which was an alternative option.

'Stevie was very calm about dying,' said Louise, 'she was accepting of it. She wanted to die at home because home was where she felt comfortable. She said she wanted to be there when things got worse.'

When things got worse.

I was not convinced. I found it difficult to believe, really, that Catherine could have wished to end her days amongst so much that was broken, fitting though it might have seemed for such a broken woman.

'I didn't know that,' I said. 'That surprises me.'

'Well, she did,' said Louise, defensively. 'Stevie was assertive. She was very clear about what she wanted.'

'So you went to the flat,' I said, wondering how anyone could think that the place I saw was fit to house a terminally sick woman. 'Did you not find it disturbing?'

'Not disturbing,' Louise answered, thoughtfully. 'Intriguing. She was a very interesting person and it just made sense, really, made sense of her. I've never been anywhere so personal in my life. It was a very personal space.'

'That's quite true,' I said.

'Had she been to Tibet?' asked Louise. 'I wasn't sure.'

'No,' I said, and I told her a bit about Catherine and India. 'You must have seen the paintings,' I said.

'Yes, she told me she was a painter,' said Louise. 'So I expected sort of large oil paintings, not what was in the flat.'

She sounded disappointed. How much more interesting for her it would have been, I thought, uncharitably, if Catherine had been a troubled genius, and Louise privy to a collection of enormous hidden canvases.

I was very perturbed. I still wasn't sure what Louise had meant when she said that she and her colleagues had done everything possible to make the flat ready for Catherine.

Whatever it was clearly didn't include making sure that Catherine had a clean bed and heating, or a working fridge.

Louise told me that the company responsible for cleaning the flat had been respectful about leaving it as it was, to a great extent. She had asked them to, because Catherine had asked her to ask them to leave the place alone.

'I can see that,' I said, 'but it was still quite a state.'

'Yes, well, they got the bathroom ready,' said Louise. 'That in itself was a lot of work. And we gave her a mobile phone, and put in an emergency cord so that she could contact someone if things were difficult.'

Difficult?

'It cost quite a lot to arrange,' said Louise, testily.

Really? I thought. So fucking what. She was worth it.

'But in the end she died in hospital,' said Louise, and she said it slightly irritably, almost as if Catherine had failed to show up at a dinner party for which the cooking had already been done. She couldn't really feel that way, surely.

'Did you go there yourself once the cleaners had been in?' I asked.

'No,' said Louise. 'I was due to, once she returned. I would have visited and seen she was okay.'

'I see,' I said, and I thought, Therein lies the problem. A cleaning company goes in to Catherine's flat, with instructions both to respect the integrity of the premises and to make them habitable and hygienic. And no one comes to explain to them exactly what that might mean. So they do what they can and someone says, 'Job done', and that's that.

What a horrible situation for Louise to have had to deal with.

'But Stevie was very clear she didn't want the flat disturbed,' Louise said, rather desperately, and I began to feel really sorry for her. 'She wasn't at all happy about our going in. I had to persuade her.'

I realised I had been a bit unfair to Louise, at least in my mind. She didn't strike me as at all dishonest, just defensive. She obviously felt bad about something but I didn't know what exactly, and I thought it unlikely she would tell me, either. By now, my arms were folded, too. She had clearly been through the bureaucratic stages required to make ready a home for a terminally sick person. That something had gone wrong was clear, and if there had been a failure it was a failure of communication. But to have been asked by Catherine to make sure her home was left virtually undisturbed whilst having the job of making it viable would have put Louise in an impossible position.

'It can't have been a very easy situation,' I said to her.

'No,' she replied.

We took the lift down to Level 2. We shook hands, and then Louise directed me to the nearest exit, which would take me back in to the heart of the city once more.

Cath

The clock on the wall was designed to look like a Polo mint. It had yellow hands and quite a loud tick. Next to it was a *Daily Telegraph* world map and an out-of-date year planner which had Partners 2000 printed across the bottom. Post-it notes on a large cork board displayed various telephone numbers: Retail Helpline; Abacus; the local police station. A post card from Bath was pinned to the board at an oblique angle: Wish you were here, it said.

On the desk was a phone, a copy of the *Bristol Evening Post*, a bottle of Lucozade, a half-eaten packet of Polos. Keys. Post. Biros. Stock orders. It was a neat office and very warm. The CCTV screen was prominently placed. They obviously had a lot of problems with shoplifters and pickpockets. I'd already had to wait because of concern for a vulnerable customer.

'Just give me a minute,' said Esther, the woman on the till who had greeted me on my arrival in the shop. 'There's an old lady out there and I'm worried about her purse.' She walked to the end of the shop and had a word with a large blond man. He nodded and went to hover near the elderly woman, stood with arms folded and face set hard, squinting, eyes scanning the shop carefully for undesirables. He looked like a Viking.

Having tipped off the security guard Esther showed me to the office behind a door at the back of the shop. The shop was not all that large but it contained most types of things you could think of wanting from a larger supermarket, and it was fairly busy.

There was a children's TV programme I used to watch as a child, called *Mr Benn*. Each week, the sober-suited, bowler-hatted Mr Benn would walk to the end of his street to visit a fancy dress shop. There, he selected a costume. The shopkeeper would direct him to a changing room where he would don, say, a suit of armour, and when he was dressed he would re-emerge, not into the shop but into a palace or on to a jousting field. He would have an adventure, at the end of which he would find himself shown to a secret or magic door. The door led inevitably back to the changing room of the shop.

Settling myself in the office I thought of Mr Benn, I don't know why. Perhaps it was being on unfamiliar territory, although I'm not the sort of person who is particularly fazed by unfamiliar territory. In fact, I like it. Perhaps it was being backstage, as it were. Perhaps it was just being there at all that was so bizarre, sitting in a decrepit part of an unfamiliar city at the back of a mini-market where my late sister bought her groceries, waiting to talk to strangers; waiting, specifically, to talk to George, the shop's proprietor.

I listened to the ticking of the Polo clock until he arrived. When he did I was relieved because his presence had an instantly reassuring quality. Burly, bearded and friendly, I guessed he was somewhere in his fifties, perhaps more.

'Hello, love,' he said, extending a hand. 'You got here okay, then.'

'No problem.'

'Magic,' said George. 'I'm sorry to have kept you waiting.'

'You didn't at all. It's very nice of you to see me.'

George's wife, Joyce, appeared.

'George, I'll bring you your sandwiches. Hello love, I'm Joyce, we spoke on the phone. Would you like a cup of tea?'

'I'd love one. Thank you.'

George shuffled some papers around on the table, pushed some things aside to make space for me.

'I didn't realise Cath had sisters or anything,' he said. 'The conversation in here was always Bristol Rovers. She was a supporter, see. If there was football on the TV, she used to try and get in to the café in West Street and watch it there. We used to call her "Rover" because of the football scarf she wore. She was even in our book as "Rover".'

'Which café was that on West Street?'

'I think it was Barry's, on the corner of Lawford's Gate.'

'Right. Well, I'll pop in and see them after you, I think.'

He looked at me.

'You look like her,' he remarked, adding quickly: 'Well, you don't look like her, obviously, but you can see a resemblance.'

'We've got the same-shaped face.'

'Yeah, that must be it.'

He shuffled the papers around a bit more.

'Sorry it's a bit messy in here,' he apologised.

I observed the neat piles.

'This isn't messy.'

He said, 'I mean, I hope I can help you. I don't know what I can tell you about Cath, really. I'm not very good with words.'

'I'm sure you are,' I reassured him. 'Tell me what you thought about Cath, what she was like.'

'Oh, she was all right, Cath was,' George replied, and despite his protestations he showed no misgivings whatever about talking. 'She was deep, mind you, you had to get to know her. She didn't give herself up very easily. If there was something you wanted to know you had to wait until she told you. There was no asking. You could make suggestions at her and wait for responses but you couldn't ask her a direct question.'

'How long had you known her?'

'When we were round the other shop was when we first met Cath. We opened in 1982 and she was one of our first customers. I used to deliver her shopping at that time, she used to buy a lot of shopping then and it was too much for her to carry so I used to pop down to her flat. I used to go to the school next door, too.'

'So you knew her for eighteen years.'

'That's right. Eighteen years we opened the doors at six o'clock in the morning and in she'd walk. She was always early and sometimes she'd stay and talk awhile and other times, she'd just come in and go out. She'd talk as the mood took her. Sometimes she'd come in, call me names, creep up behind me and slap me on the back of the head, just playful, friendly.'

George paused.

'Mind you,' he went on, 'you could go a couple of weeks and she didn't want to talk at all. I might wind her up a bit and she'd say, 'I don't feel like it today. Leave me alone.' But that was as far as it got, it never got nasty. Sometimes, she'd hang around outside. She'd stand outside for hours some mornings, just on her own without ever saying anything, and then she'd be back to normal again. I used to wonder if it was the medication she was on.'

Joyce had reappeared with George's sandwiches and my tea.

'How old was your sister?' she asked.

'Forty-seven.'

'Oh, we thought she was about that age, didn't we, George.'

'Yeah,' said George, nodding. 'Did she ever travel?'

'Yes,' I replied.

'Because she used to talk about Tibet, Nepal and India a lot,' he said. 'She used to talk about the Dalai Lama, nothing that you could say was a conversation, just snippets. Every now and again it might crop up and you'd think, Well, she's obviously been somewhere, and you didn't really like to ask. And she'd obviously had a good education, you could tell.'

'Yes,' said Joyce. 'And we did wonder about her travelling because of what she used to say, didn't we. We used to wonder if it was a flight of fancy.'

'Yeah,' said George, 'but she just knew too much to be making it up.'

'That's right,' said Joyce. 'She did.'

'The Dalai Lama seemed to have played some big part in her life,' George continued. 'And whenever I've been going on holiday, she'd say, "Where are you going, George?" and I'd tell her and she'd say, "Go to Nepal and Tibet and see the foothills of the Himalayas." She really made it sound nice.'

He took a bite of his sandwich.

Joyce said, 'Do you know, thinking about her age, she didn't look any different now from how she did then.'

'No,' affirmed George, 'she never changed. That's why you couldn't really put an age on her. Mind you, she was always together, always. You wouldn't look at her and say she was out of the way.'

'No, you wouldn't,' Joyce agreed.

'You get a few come through these doors that are,' said George, 'but she was never like that. She was always washed, hair combed. She had a big zip-up brown leather jacket she used to wear.'

'That's right,' said Joyce.

'Cath was as straight as they come, too,' he insisted, 'which is more than you can say about a lot around this way. She was as honest as the day was long, really honest. Right to the end, she told me she was ill but I didn't know how serious, she didn't go into it, but she made sure that the bill was paid up. It was hardly anything in the end, you're talking maybe £6 or £7, but she came all the way down to pay it. However short she was, she always paid.'

'That's good,' I said.

'What Cath used to do, a few times the bill got over the top and she'd say, "Would you write me out a bill and send it to my mother?" And I'd write the bill out, she'd send it off, and back would come a cheque from your mother. It was never really a problem. I'd sometimes say, "A bit high this week, Cath," and she'd say, "What if I don't have the food? I can get that elsewhere." So she'd buy the tobacco and I suppose she went to the café and they kept her with food. She never struck me that she was going hungry but we wouldn't have let that happen anyway. We'd always give her a sandwich in the morning. She'd come in, she'd say, "Can I have a sandwich?" "Yeah, course you can." We used to make it especially, in the end.'

Joyce made for the door.

'You'll have to excuse me,' she said. 'I'd better get back.'

George nodded.

'We used to have a fellow come in here,' George gestured backwards towards the shop with his thumb, 'he pinched the cheese. We knew he was pinching it and when he came to the counter I'd just take a few extra bob off what he bought and he paid for it that way. He was never a real thief, it was just circumstances, I suppose. He'd got that way. And I mean, a piece of cheese and a sandwich is not very much, is it. It helps.'

He added, 'I did send Cath a few bob when she was in the hospital because she'd phoned and asked for her tobacco and I thought she wouldn't be able to get out to collect her money or anything; so I sent a few fivers up there and every-thing was paid back, everything. She was so honest it wasn't true. She never took advantage. I wish I was better with words, really, I could sort of get it over to you differently.'

I said, 'You're getting it over perfectly.'

We drank our tea together and George made some progress with his sandwich.

'Did she strike you as lonely?' I asked.

'She struck me as not lonely but a loner,' George answered, 'which is a different thing, isn't it.'

'Yes, I agree.'

'I think she was quite content in her own company but sort of spent her life on her own. There are people that are that way. Although I did see her with someone else, not recently, but there was a fellow that used to go around with her a bit, must have been two or three years ago. I don't know his name but he was with her for about a year and they always came in together. Whether there was anything there, I don't know. He used to share her tobacco. I think he was a street person because I've seen him since, I've seen him recently, to be honest. But they just weren't together after a bit. It might just be that they passed the time of day together, I don't really know, but I never thought of her as bothering with men and that sort of thing, to be honest.'

'No, I don't think she did.'

I considered asking George more about this elusive companion of my elusive sister, and then I thought about the fact that he lived on the streets and George didn't know his name. While that may not have made it impossible to find him, it certainly made it pretty difficult, unless I hung about with George in his shop for days on end. I wondered about asking George to ask the man to get in touch with me, should he see him. Some chance, I thought.

'There was a few she didn't get on with very well,' George continued. 'There was a fellow that come in, Craig I think his name is. I don't really know him very well but he's got two kids, he's by himself, and what I've heard is that he used to live next to her years ago and they didn't get on then, apparently. She'd follow him up the road and call him a couple of names, you know, shout after him.'

'Did they ever get into fights?'

'Not that I know of, no.'

'Because I wouldn't put it past her.'

'No,' said George. 'I know what you mean. She always used to stand her ground, she didn't buckle down to him. He's a big man as well. He's a nasty piece of work. But she wasn't. She came across as a nice person. She was a nice person.'

He paused.

'I don't know if it's strange to say but I liked her. She was just one of those people that you like.'

'Well, I imagine she was very fond of you,' I said. 'I think coming here probably meant a lot to her because she didn't find it very easy to have close friendships with people. I think the friendship she had with you was very important. You know, she could come in when it suited her; she could stand outside if she liked and it wasn't a problem. No one hassled her.'

George said, 'Must have been long days for her, when you think about it.'

I had thought about it, often. I remember wondering, when bored in lessons at school, what my older sister was doing at that precise minute. I remember looking out of the window during maths, a window that afforded a very good view of the Downs beyond, and trying to imagine where she might be.

'Yeah, I think they were. And long nights, too.'

'You'd never see her after dinner hour,' said George. 'Afternoons she was never about. Where she went, I don't know.'

I said, 'I think she probably slept, though I'm not sure. I

don't think she slept very well at night.'

'Yeah,' said George, 'come to think of it, I seem to remember she listened to her music at night. She came in one day with a big stereo she'd got somewhere and we got her some headphones for it because some neighbours had complained about the noise.'

'She liked music,' I said. 'I picked up her collection from the flat and she had jazz and rock and classical and folk; all sorts. In our family there was always a lot of music. And she played the piano.'

'Did she? She struck me as that sort.'

I wondered what sort.

'You know,' George continued. 'Cultured.'

I remembered there was something I'd wanted to know.

'Did she buy a newspaper, George?'

'Occasionally, yeah. I don't think it was very often but when she did it would be like *The Times* or *Telegraph*, big papers. Now I think of it,' he added, 'it was always *The Times*.'

She read *The Times*. I was very taken aback by that. I hadn't expected it, I don't know why. I wondered whether she'd ever seen any of the book reviews that I wrote for the paper. At one stage, I wrote two a month. I used to love reviewing. In the days before my children were born, when I was writing my own books full- instead of part-time and I had more time in general, reviewing other people's was very interesting. I wondered whether Catherine had seen the interviews with me on the features pages when my own books were published. I wondered whether she'd seen the photograph in the paper of me on my wedding day, printed alongside an article I'd written about Robert Runcie, the friend who had valiantly given our wedding address the day after beginning heavy chemotherapy treatment for the cancer that eventually killed him.

Probably not. But who knows?

I thought, So near and yet so far.

'And I shouldn't be saying this,' George was saying, 'but the top shelf books, they used to disgust her. She used to really have a go at me about selling those. But there's a demand, isn't there, and you can't just ignore it. She used to say, "You should never have that kind of thing on the shelves." She was prudish really, because they were all in covers, it wasn't like there was anything showing. But she didn't like it.'

'No, I can imagine that.'

George fiddled idly with a biro on the desk.

'Was it the illness that made her a loner, do you think?' he asked.

'Yes, I do. Mainly the illness, anyway.'

He nodded.

'But I think you're probably right that she wasn't lonely,' I agreed. 'After all, she had a lot of people that she knew and saw. I was talking with Father McKay about her and he told me that he used to pay her annual subscription to Amnesty International. That was really nice of him.'

'She used to go and see the one before Father McKay, Father O'Brien. She used to go down and sit with him quite a bit.'

'They were obviously very good to her.'

'Yeah,' said George, 'but then she was one of the characters in the area. Everybody knew her. I think a lot of people just knew her in passing, you know, because I'd be driving here to the shop and she'd be right down the other end of Station Road, walking. She walked miles. And if she saw you she was always waving, you know, making a big thing of it.'

'Right.'

'But then she was just one of many around here,' George

explained. 'To be honest, if you spend a week in this place you don't notice that kind of thing in the end. You don't, because there's so many that are like it, there's so many people with - I was going to say "with an illness", but some of what you see is just people living on their own and they mutter to themselves because they've got nobody else.'

'It's a pretty mixed area, isn't it.'

'Oh it is, it is,' George agreed. 'I don't know if it's the same where you come from but it's eye-opening in this area. Some of it's self-inflicted: drugs, most of it, these days. I've moved out of the area now but I moved here first in '69, got married and lived in those flats across the road. The flats were brand new when I moved there and it was luxury to us because we moved out of houses with gas fires and gaslights. They've turned into slums since, really seedy places. Most of the city's going the same way. There was shootings last weekend.'

'Were there?'

'Yeah. Two men shot dead.'

'Here?' I asked, and George nodded.

'They picked them up round the corner, then took them up on the Downs and shot them dead.'

'Drugs, right?'

'You bet your life on it.'

'Terrible,' I said.

George shook his head.

'Yeah. And there was a shooting about two weeks ago, just along the road again. It's amazing. I spent all my life down here and it's only in the last ten years it's got like it has now.'

I looked at George's second, untouched sandwich.

'You'd better finish your lunch,' I said. 'I've kept you talking.'

But George's mind wasn't on food.

'It's a shame,' he said, shaking his head. 'A real shame, Cath going like that.'

'Yes.'

'That was too young to die, wasn't it. Too young. When you see how some of them abuse themselves around here.'

'Yes, it was too young.'

George sighed.

'I'd like to have been to her funeral,' he said, and there was sharp regret in his voice, 'but there was no one to ask. Well, I'll be honest with you, I did have your mum's phone number but I didn't know what you knew. And I thought, well, it was Cath's wishes, wasn't it. Being on her own was what she wanted, so you wanted to respect it. She never said if she'd told your mum she was ill, so I thought it was best left alone. But there was no one you could go to and say, "Just how ill is she?" When I did pluck up the nerve, I phoned the hospital and they said she'd been moved to Oncology, and I phoned there and they said she was okay. So I left it a few more weeks and I phoned again and they said she'd died. In between that time, she had come down and paid all her bills up. I suppose she was out of hospital for a bit. It must have been a real effort for her to come down here.'

'Did she tell you that she was ill?' I asked.

'She said something to Joyce about it, and if she was that ill then, it was very brave of her to carry on, very brave the way she accepted it. She said it was a cancer she had and she said, "There's some they can do something about and some they can't. And it's my luck", she said, "I've got one of those they can't." '

George sighed.

'It must be a terrible thing to accept,' he mused. 'We were never really that sure how ill she was. She did say, "I'm very ill" to me but you couldn't reach her to ask how ill. There were limits and you couldn't get personal or get beyond the limit, if you know what I mean.

'It's like with the sandwich,' he said, expansively. 'We'd say to her, "Want this, Cath? Otherwise it's going in the bin." That way, she'd take it. But if she thought you'd made it for her especially, it was a different matter. There was ways of approaching her and you had to know her to understand that, didn't you. I mean, she wasn't the easiest sort of person. You knew what she wanted you to know. It was as simple as that, really.'

'I know what you mean.'

George looked a little embarrassed.

'Of course, here's me telling you what your own sister's like and that's not right,' he said, apologetically. 'I mean, what I'm really trying to say is, I've never met you before though I've spoke to your mum, but I don't see that any of you acted wrongly because I know that much about Cath. I knew how she was. I knew she wanted to be left alone.'

'She did, yes. But this was obviously a very important place to her, your shop.'

George looked pleased at the affirmation.

'She rang me from the hospital a couple of times,' he said. I was surprised.

'Did she?'

'Yeah. And I sent that tobacco up to her, stuck it in the post.'

'That was really nice of you. She would have appreciated that.'

'Yeah, she did smoke a bit,' he said, drily.

'I'm afraid that's what probably did for her in the end.'

George nodded sadly.

I suddenly wondered about drink. I had no memory of Catherine drinking anything at all but I asked him, 'Did she ever buy alcohol?'

'I've never known her buy alcohol. No, never.'

'I don't think she drank at all.'

'No. Cuppa Soups and noodles she seemed to exist on. Cream crackers. She'd come and do her shopping Thursday mornings and the bill was always paid the following Tuesday. You could set the time by her. And she never paid a bill unless I was here myself to take it.'

George paused.

'Towards the end,' he said, 'she'd very often come in and ask for a glass of water to take her Nurofen. She had suffered with toothache for a long time and she had that put right and then she just kept coming for the Nurofen. She had boxes and boxes of Nurofen.'

'They're expensive, Nurofen.'

'Cor, not half! I used to tell her that. I used to say to her, "Go and get a prescription. You get the prescription free." '

'Perhaps she didn't want to admit to her doctor how ill she felt,' I suggested.

'But she knew herself, didn't she.'

'Yes, she knew. She found a lump but she didn't say anything for a long time. She was scared, didn't want to deal with it.'

'I can understand that,' said George.

'I can, too.'

'The tendency is, "don't look", isn't it,' George said. 'The other thing with the Nurofen was, I don't think cash was a very important part of her life, to be honest. Of course, you have to exist, you have to live, but I think she had what she wanted. Whatever she had in her pocket, she would still have lived the same way.'

'She never struck you as wanting more?' I enquired.

'No.' George was emphatic. 'She never struck me as bitter about anything, to be honest with you.'

'Or depressed?'

'Or depressed, no. The life she had she accepted. I mean, she'd obviously come from better, so it must have been hard to be able to accept things like that but she was quite content.'

All this time, contemplating the kind, decent man before me, I'd been wondering how I might raise the subject of Steve. Had George known about Steve but been too polite to say so? And would he be shocked, if he hadn't known, to find out? I figured not a lot would shock George but you never quite know with people. I certainly didn't want to be the person to shatter the image of someone he had liked and looked after so well. I didn't want him to be upset or, worse, repulsed.

'Did she ever ask,' I began and then faltered, momentarily losing confidence in my enquiry. 'Did she ever ask you to call her anything different from Cath?'

'No. But I have heard people say that. I can't remember what the name was now.'

I took a deep breath.

'Steve?' I ventured.

'Steve, yeah, that's right. I've heard people say that. I mean, once she did say to me, "Don't call me Cath." She said, "Don't call me Cath, I'm not a woman," but that was as far as it went, just the one time. And I didn't ask. You never ask, it was never anybody else's business. Anyway, these days that happens a lot, doesn't it. I mean, I've got a daughter, I've never seen her in a dress. She's sixteen years old and I've never seen her in a dress! She just won't wear one. It's just jeans. So really, Cath never struck me as anything out the way in that way. I suppose years ago you thought, Women in skirts and men in trousers, but that's long gone now.'

I sighed with relief.

'So to you she was Cath.'

'Yeah, always Cath. And she never appeared any different to me. She was always the same.'

I looked at the Polo clock. I had taken up enough of George's day.

'I must go, George. It's been incredibly kind of you to give up your time like this.'

'It's nothing. I don't feel I've been any help at all, though. I wish I could tell you more.'

'You've been a great help.'

I gathered my things together and we made our way back in to the shop.

'Though there was one thing,' said George. 'I suppose she got more, not playful, that's not the word, but less serious, as I got to know her. When she talked, when we first knew her, it was just about the business we were doing, but then the football came along and opened all sorts of doors. You could really get to her through that, and she had a good sense of humour, I tell you. She knew how to wind me up and some mornings it was a real slanging match, but it was always fun. Back at one Christmas, she said, "I'm going to get you something," and she came back with a Rovers scarf, they were her team, not mine. She also brought me a couple of paintings that she'd done. It was a guardsman, one of them, the Mounted Guards that stand at Horseguards Parade. I think she had that back after; I know there was one where she said, "I wish I hadn't given you that, I want it."'

I said, 'She loved to paint. She'd done a lot of paintings.'

'Had she?'

'Yes, we found a lot in her flat. Thousands. Literally thousands.'

'Cor,' said George. 'Thousands!'

I looked around the shop. A man nearby was examining a tin of something. Another, younger man, was buying a newspaper. An elderly woman in a thick coat was shuffling slowly towards us down a side aisle.

'Did she ever talk to other customers at all?'

'Not really, no,' said George. 'Come to think of it, though,' he remembered, 'Valerie who works here said that Cath used to like her dog, Trixie. Sometimes Valerie would tie Trixie to the baskets at the end and I remember Cath down there, talking to the dog. She was also very nice to elderly people if she met them in the shop. A Mrs Tyler used to come in here and Cath would always make a point, if she was here, of pushing her way in up the queue and filling Mrs Tyler's bag up, to save her packing herself.'

I said, 'I think she preferred animals to people.'

'Yeah,' said George, 'can't say I really blame her.'

I realised I was suddenly pretty hungry.

I said, 'I'll just get a sandwich, if that's okay,' and I went to select one, only to find that I was incapable of making a decision. I stood for an inordinately long time in front of the chiller, my mind a curious blank, gazing at bacon and egg, ham and cheese, cheese and pickle, chicken, prawns. I couldn't think straight, couldn't think at all. I wondered what sort of sandwich Catherine had liked best. I picked up a prawn sandwich. Then I thought of the giant hoovers that are used to harvest seafood, machines that simultaneously inhale every form of seabed flora and fauna, so I put the prawn sandwich back and took a cheese one. But I don't much care for cheese, so I swapped back to the prawn after all and picked up a bottle of mineral water. Get a grip, girl, I told myself. At the counter, I picked up a banana and handed some money to George.

He shook his head and gently pushed my hand away.

'Oh no, George, really, you've been so kind, let me pay.'

'No way,' he said. 'It's on us.'

'Oh, George.'

'It's the last thing we can do for Cath,' he said. 'Feed up her sister.'

He handed me a caramel bar, to add to my lunch. There were tears in his eyes.

And there and then I realised something. I realised that in every village, every town, every city and every country, there are people like George doing kind, decent, selfless things simply because to do those things is right. They do not live in active pursuit of justice and parity and their intention and influence is not dramatic. But every day, they are lifting elderly relations out of bed, collecting shopping, giving lifts, sharing cups of tea, passing the time of day. I thought how easy it is to expose yourself, via the news if nothing else, to everything that is disgusting and heartbreaking about the world; and how difficult it is to remember that for all the wanton acts of violence there are unsung acts of generosity. For all the evil out there, there is warmth and compassion. A cold child starves: another is tucked up in bed with a full belly. A blind man is beaten up in his home: another is visited by a neighbour, who reads to him.

It isn't a simple question of balance. No one could be so naïve as to believe that. Kindness shown in one place doesn't touch someone subjected to violence in another, and Catherine's breakfast didn't make any difference to someone else who was hungry. Daily, trust is wrecked and lives ruined: repair is not always possible and atonement rare. The world turns and surely, repeatedly, humanity disgraces itself. Yet there is hope. At least, there is if you believe that the good that is done can serve as a significant compensation for the bad. If so, perhaps an act of neglect elsewhere was negated by each sandwich George made for Catherine in Bristol. That is fanciful, maybe, but it makes it easier to remember that for weakness, deceit, self-interest, cowardice and wickedness there is always consideration, mercy, altruism, compassion and moral courage.

It was written on Catherine's wall and the words made sense to me now: *Thank you, George.*

'You'll come back again, won't you,' said George, 'whenever you're in the area.'

'I will. Most certainly.'

'You're off to the café now, then?'

'Well, I'm going to the drop-in centre around the corner first because Richard McKay told me he thinks she went there sometimes. But I'll go and see if I have any luck at the café, too. Barry's on the corner of Lawford's Gate and West Street, right?'

'That's right, and if you're going to the drop-in centre you can take a short cut across the grass opposite the shop if you want. It's not far.'

'I'll do that.'

''Bye then, love,' said George. 'Go carefully.'

Dropping In

I took George's route across the grass, the one that ran between the flats in which he had once lived. He was right that they had seen far better days. En route, I ate my sandwich. There was almost no one around, although two policemen walked past me. One of them smiled, and I smiled back. Catherine hated police. She always thought they were about to arrest her.

On the way to the Methodist Centre I caught sight of Barry's café. I thought about dropping in but decided it should wait. I was due at the Methodist Centre and I was already fifteen minutes late. George had spent much more time with me than I'd expected.

A couple of minutes' walk from the café, the centre was situated in a tall, narrow building that was part of a terrace of Victorian houses. Most of them were now flats, in poor condition. I rang the doorbell and waited. The views each way were bleak: buildings in need of attention, some boarded up; litter on the street and nothing green in sight. A cleared site opposite, plus evidence of recent road-widening, implied that a certain amount of building was about to take place although whether this would lead to positive regeneration of the immediate area was another matter. Making it less than depressing was going to take a hell of a lot more than some extra housing.

A young man opened the door. He was around twenty years old, wearing a baggy wool jersey and Jesus-creeper sandals. His hair was blond and slightly ruffled.

I explained who I was all over again.

'I've come to see Richard Barrett, the minister here,' I said. 'I spoke to him on the phone last week. He knows I'm coming. I'm a bit late, I'm afraid.'

'Ah,' beamed the man. 'Well, I'm Joe. I'm a volunteer. Come on in.' He extended his arm upwards and behind him to indicate a steep staircase. 'Welcome.'

We walked up three flights of stairs, passing rooms that would once have been bedrooms. Now, they were offices and informal meeting rooms. There were cardboard boxes on the landings and notice boards on the walls. The carpet was hard-wearing, industrial, no longer domestic.

A middle-aged man was standing at the top of the stairs talking to a younger man wearing a stripy T-shirt and combat trousers. He was tall and imposing.

'A-ha,' he said, as Joe and I appeared. 'Is this who I think it is?'

But he didn't say it with any humour. He was suspicious of me, or so it seemed. I couldn't blame him, really. What did he know about me?

'Depends what you're thinking,' I replied. 'I'm Mary, Cathy Loudon's sister. How do you do. I'm terribly sorry to be late. It's my fault.'

'Are you late?' he asked, vaguely. 'Well, I've got to go early anyway. I can give you a few minutes.'

We shook hands and exchanged some pleasantries but there was wariness on both sides, or perhaps the wariness was mine alone. Perhaps he was always like this, professional, distant. Maybe I was just tired. It had felt like a long day so far.

'We'll be best off in the dining room, I think,' said Richard, and he led me into a room with tables, chairs and a serving counter that divided the room from the kitchen beyond. The atmosphere was very smoky. A radio was on in the kitchen and a man was talking loudly in another room nearby. There was something about the urgency in his voice that registered with me. It reminded me a little of Catherine. He didn't sound well. Someone else was playing the guitar and singing, 'Everybody Hurts'.

Richard didn't have a lot of time, he made that clear once more.

'I've got to lock up in ten minutes.'

I offered to go away.

'No, no. Have a seat.'

I sat but my hackles rose. It wasn't Richard's fault. It was an automatic response to something in his tone I couldn't quite determine. I think it was the faint air of clericalism and although it was faint it got up my nose. When I was very young – eighteen years old – I met through someone else a whole lot of clergy and found them, like any group, to be very mixed. Most were absolutely fine; good people with a decent purpose. Some were outstanding, some dull. But a few were unspeakable, mostly because they were desperately insecure. In fact, the insecure were the worst because they were very often vicious while the dullards were simply pompous; and some were both so vapid and so patronising it was farcical.

However, one characteristic shared by these less-than-average clergy was their tendency to lean over the drawings of small children, the beds of the sick, or the thresholds of local houses and say in exactly the same tone of wheedling condescension: 'And how's it all going? Oh, well done, you!' They would chirrup to parishioners returning to church congregations after absences caused by anything from holidays to marriage breakdowns to chemotherapy: 'Back with us all? Marvellous. Well done, you!' They were the sort for whom 'Well done, you!' and 'Have you come far?' seemed to cover almost everything from birth to marriage to death, everything, that is, except for their inability to talk to people properly.

A man emerged from the kitchen to ask Richard a question about the tea urn that sat on the serving counter between the kitchen and dining room. Richard answered perfectly easily and agreeably. I composed myself. Steady on, I thought: give the poor bloke a chance. There are a lot of thoughtful men and women of faith out there. There are a lot of people who are trying hard. Richard was almost certainly one of them. If I felt rather raw that afternoon it was not his problem. It was mine.

'Really,' he said, 'Trudy's the one you should probably be speaking to. She's been here longer than I have. She told me that Cathy apparently liked being here if there were small children, in the family room next door.'

'Oh.' I was surprised. 'That's interesting.'

'And the fact that Trudy was quite confident about her being there is quite interesting too,' Richard pointed out.

I hadn't thought of that. Catherine's edginess might well have been off-putting to anyone supervising a group of young children.

He added, 'Trudy also remarked that she found Cathy was something of a perfectionist, very particular about things. They had to be done in the right way, meet her approval. I'm not sure whether Trudy did her washing for her, I've a feeling perhaps she did. Trudy, because she's near the laundry, often did washing for people.'

So this was where Catherine washed her clothes. I had been wondering. I'd forgotten to ask whether there were facilities at the flats where she lived, though I guessed there must have been.

'Cathy used to pop up and see me occasionally in the office,' Richard continued. 'She would not spend time really happily in the day room with lots of other people but if she could find a private space with you, she would. She would suddenly appear and suddenly disappear is my memory of her.'

He paused, then said: 'It was quite intense, what she told me. She gave me an account of some of her life which was pretty harrowing, if it was true.'

I waited for more but it was not forthcoming.

'I remember she went off,' he remarked, instead, 'with a tape of ours. She wanted to borrow a tape of Christmas carols, interestingly, which she must still have.'

'I may have them,' I said. 'I've got some of her tapes.'

'Oh, I don't need it back,' answered Richard, 'but it's just interesting that she was very insistent she wanted to borrow something about Christmas. This is a couple of years ago now,' he added.

I wondered why he thought it interesting that Catherine should have wanted to borrow something about Christmas. Did he think that Christmas wouldn't matter to her? Did he imagine that she was too mad to enjoy it, or did he simply assume that with its connotations of family togetherness, she would have been unlikely to want to celebrate the festival? Did her wish to listen to carols indicate to him that she might, after all, have some religious leanings that he had not himself detected? I didn't ask him. I didn't have the energy somehow.

'In general,' he went on, 'I found conversations with her difficult. Somehow she seemed to be pleased to have someone who would listen and that's what we try and do here but conversations as such were not easy. I hadn't seen her for a while, either. Most recently I would have seen her on the street and just given her a wave, and she would always sort of duck her head and wave back, but I don't know why she didn't come in so much of late.'

'She was ill,' I suggested, 'and she did know she was ill.
That might explain it. I get the impression that she with-
drew from a lot of things at the end of her life.'

Richard nodded.

'She had told Trudy that she was ill,' he said, 'Trudy knew
she had cancer.'

He broke off to greet someone who entered the room in
haste and then departed again almost as quickly. A woman
called up the stairs and a man answered. A door slammed.

'Hmm,' he said, distractedly, 'yes.' He turned back to me.
'She was one of those shadowy figures that does come
around and evidently feels relatively at home here.' He
paused. 'The sort who often doesn't feel at home in other
places.' He paused again. 'That's all I can say really.'

That was all he could say. I don't know what I had been
hoping for but it wasn't what Richard had described: 'one
of those shadowy figures'. I gazed at a notice on the walls
about remembering not to leave the urn too long at boiling
point. I could see why. Condensation from the urn had
spread throughout the dining room and I was aware of the
slight damp tackiness of the table before me. No, I had been
hoping for an individual, someone more substantially fleshed
out than this ethereal presence which even now eluded me.
Even now, when I was sitting in a building Catherine had
visited, with a man she had known, I felt no closer to her.
Just as George had animated my sister, Richard had rendered
her indistinguishable once more.

'Obviously it is nice if, at a certain stage of her life, it was
helpful to her to come here,' he said. He was attempting to
be helpful. He was trying, I could see, to provide sustenance
where in reality there was little to be had.

I understood then that I could not fairly explain any
failure of mine to find Catherine in the Methodist Centre by
feeling disappointed in this person who had, after all, agreed

to meet me in the first place. If Catherine's personality and character was obscure to him it was hardly surprising. It didn't make him culpable. I began to realise that it was too much to expect other people to reveal my sister to me. If I caught a glimpse of her from time to time, as I had with George Jefferies and Richard McKay, then I should be grateful. A glimpse, after all, was more than I had had for quite some time. And an occasional glimpse was all that Richard himself had had, which didn't leave him much to offer me.

'I'm sure it was helpful to her,' I said, hoping that I sounded sincere. I felt I needed to make it up to him somehow, this lack of the sister I was seeking. 'Do you know, by the way, if she came in here and had lunch much?'

'I don't think so.'

'Because when I first heard about her coming here I thought, Ah, probably she went so she could eat.'

'That's not my memory of it,' Richard shook his head. 'I wouldn't swear to it but I would have said that would have been too public for her; although there was a whole period before I came here and other workers probably knew her over that period. I suspect she has had a long association with the place.'

I said, 'She may have done but she moved around a bit. She also went to the charity run by the Cyrenians in years gone by. I know she ate there. Do you know them at all?'

'Well, we have contact, yes,' said Richard, non-committally. 'The staff there will have changed a lot. That's always the trouble with a place like here, and like there.'

He looked at his watch.

I said, 'This is inconvenient for you. I'll go.'

'It's all right,' said Richard.

I felt a bit lost. I smiled, lamely.

'Is there anything else you want to know?' Richard asked.

'No,' I said. 'I mean, yes. Well, anything really. But you're busy. Really, I should go.' And I began to gather my coat from the chair beside me.

Richard raised a hand in an attitude that said, Hang on a minute. I put my coat down. I decided that the effect on other people of his height and stature must have helped Richard over the years to keep his gestures to a bare minimum.

'Well, what kind of things?' he asked.

I took a deep breath.

'When you said,' I began, 'I mean, I quite appreciate there are some things you probably don't want to repeat because they're private to you and her, so I wouldn't dream of asking you to do that. But is there anything about the difficult stuff in her life that you would care to repeat?'

'Oh, right,' said Richard, in precisely the sort of tone someone might use to say, 'Oh, is that all?' 'Well, what she spoke about was having travelled abroad and being in . . . I forget whether it was Thailand or China or where.'

He looked at his watch again.

'India,' I said.

'India, was it? She talked about having been the subject of a lot of persecution and having been put in jail, and having suffered a great deal. I mean, it was all slightly bizarre and I wasn't sure what to make of it.'

'No,' I said, 'that's everybody's reaction. I mean, nobody knows whether it actually happened or not. My feeling is that it ceases to matter actually because for her it was real. We just don't know. She was very ill.'

'Yes,' Richard agreed. 'My sense was that there was a swing between moods and that sometimes she could come in quite high, quite bubbly, quite excited, but at other times very low and very distressed. We saw both.'

'Did she ever mention that she had a family?'

'I don't recall.'

'I see.'

He said, with some dispatch, 'She just seemed a very isolated and lonely person and you were happy that she felt able to come in here.'

'Right.'

He sounded so conclusive, as if Catherine were just one of many people like her. From his point of view, I suppose, she was. There are Catherines everywhere, and some of the Bristol Catherines pitch up daily at the Methodist Centre. But I was only looking for one. Mine.

I gazed hopelessly around the room. The guitar was still being played next door, a Leonard Cohen song now, 'Suzanne'. I should have been happy that Catherine was able to come here, too, but I didn't feel very happy about anything at that moment. Leonard Cohen wasn't helping; a fine musician, possibly, but a moody songster.

'I'm going to have to close in a minute,' said Richard, and this time I put on my coat and stood up. A man looking at his watch and a woman looking for her dead sister do not belong together. Richard had somewhere to go that was real and present: I had someone to find who wasn't. There was no moral advantage inherent in either position but there was tension between the two.

I said, 'I'm sorry to have come at an awkward time but I really appreciate your taking the time to see me.'

I extended my hand.

Richard shook it and smiled.

'Not at all,' he said. 'I just have to close, that's all.'

Emerging on to the main road outside I inhaled air free of stale smoke and sad songs. To my right and across the road was Barry's café.

The door to the café was open. I walked in. It was quiet

and currently empty of customers but a young man and older woman were behind the counter. The woman was scooping mayonnaise and egg from a large container into a smaller one. The man was writing something on a notepad. He looked up and brushed a straggle of hair from his forehead with his forearm.

'Can I help you, love?'

I explained who I was. I described Catherine.

He shook his head solemnly.

'I'm very sorry,' he said. 'I didn't ever know anyone like that. Ask my mother.'

The woman too was at a loss.

She said, 'Ask my other son, he's here in the mornings.'

'I'm only here today,' I said. 'I'm leaving pretty soon.'

'Oh dear,' she lamented. 'I'm sorry.'

'Have you tried the café two doors down?' asked the man. 'She might have been there, because I'm sure I would have known her if she came here. Maybe the person who told you she did got mixed up.'

'Maybe they did. That's a good idea, I'll try the other place. Thank you.'

The pair of them smiled kindly, in unison.

'And where is your sister now?' the man enquired, politely.

I told them that Catherine was dead.

The woman inclined her head.

She said, with great formality, 'I offer you my condolences.'

What Kind of
Sister Are You?

The café was spacious, airless and warm. The tables were made of moulded orange plastic, the chairs fixed to the floor. Each table was furnished with salt and pepper and a stand-up plastic menu. There was a bank of slot machines at the back of the room. A middle-aged woman with dyed black hair and a younger man wearing a large, soft brown leather jacket were wrestling them into position. This was taking them a long time. When they had finished, panting and sweating slightly, they stood and surveyed the room's altered geography.

'Bingo's too big,' the woman remarked, indicating a machine near the counter.

'Yeah, it is for in here,' agreed the man.

He turned slightly and noticed me.

'Sorry,' he said, 'do you want to go ahead and order?'

'It's okay,' I replied, 'I'll wait.'

After more discussion about the bingo machine the woman turned to me. Personally, I thought they should have spaced the machines out a bit. They looked uninviting in a long line.

I asked her about Catherine. She didn't know.

'We've just bought the place,' she explained. 'We've only been here four weeks. But Victor might know. He's a regular, been coming for years.'

She pointed her finger towards a man sitting at a table next to the wall. All of his features, but particularly his neck, were thick and bulbous. His purple-skinned face was lumpy and mottled. He was wearing a heavy gold chain and his shirt was unbuttoned almost to his navel. His stomach spilled over his waistband, concealing his groin, and rested upon the tops of his thighs.

I reminded myself that it is medieval to judge people by their physiognomy. I approached the table and very carefully and politely explained my purpose to Victor.

He was eating sausage and chips and drinking coke.

'She was your sister?'

His voice was raspy.

'That's right.'

He looked me up and down.

'You got a photograph?'

I bridled. 'No.'

'And she was your sister?'

'That's right. She was my sister.'

He wheezed uncomfortably. He was chewing on a fat chip.

'She could've been going under an alias. And you'd never know, would you. I mean, if you got no photo, how do you know what she was like?'

'She did, actually,' I replied, curtly. 'She did have an alias. She was also known as Steve.'

He didn't flinch.

'Never heard of her,' he grunted, and he turned to the woman behind the counter.

'What about that other one?' he demanded. 'That one who gave you trouble.'

'Pauline.'

'Yeah. She was a bloke.'

'Yeah, but she had long hair.'

He looked at me again, up and down.

'You ain't got no photo?'

'No.'

'She's your sister and you ain't got no photo?'

'No. Not a recent one.'

'What kind of sister are you if you ain't got no photo?'

I apologised silently to Catherine. Why should a cat, a dog and Victor have life and Catherine no life at all?

I took my leave, as calmly as I could.

Chip suspended on fork, Victor shouted towards the door: 'So what, she die in an accident or something?'

Outside Barry's café, two doors down, was a shiny black cab, slightly different in design from the usual kind. There was no one inside it.

A man's voice called out: 'You want a cab, love?'

The taxi driver was sitting just inside the door of Barry's café. There was an empty coffee cup next to his elbow. He was reading the *Sun* newspaper.

He drove me to Bristol Temple Meads station. The cab was very swish indeed, shiny and new, as capacious as an ocean liner.

'Great cab,' I said.

'Everyone likes this cab. Mercedes. Forty K. I'm still halfway through paying it off. It cost me two K this year.'

I asked if he'd been busy recently.

'I have, though I went home last night after two jobs feeling ill. Still feel a bit rough but I'm okay. I'm diabetic. I say to all the girls, "You come with me in my cab. I'm safe, I'm on the pill." '

He swept into the station concourse and two young women flagged him down.

'You see,' he chuckled, 'Here they are to prove it.'

I handed over the fare.

'Thanks for the ride. Hope you feel better soon.'

'No problem, sweetheart. You go carefully now.'

'I will.'

The two women sprung into the cab.

'Brown's, please,' they chorused in happy, sing-song voices. Girls just out of the office, ready to kick off their shoes.

The driver pivoted the cab around one hundred and eighty degrees.

'Righto,' he said, 'Brown's it is.'

What Kind of
Sister Was I?

Unfamiliar with what Catherine liked to eat.
   Didn't know she read the newspaper.
   No concept of how she spent her time.
   Unaware she loved football.
   No idea her name was Steve.

So it's not an unreasonable question, really: what kind of
sister are you? And the answer is that I was a sister without
access to the privy chamber of her sibling's larder, bedroom
or soul. I was, in short, a sister in obscurity.

   The irony is that for years Catherine was the one who
looked that way to me, with her locked door and locked
mind and her uneasy relationship with the world outside
them. She was the one on the outskirts of life. She was the
one in the dark, or so I had thought. But it was *trompe
l'oeil*, a trick of the light. She knew where we were and what
we were doing because we told her. We sent news and photographs. We told her when babies were born and dogs died.
If anyone was in obscurity, we were. She was simply out of
reach.

   Obscurity is an inauspicious state. Not knowing something about someone to whom you are related puts you at
a distinct disadvantage in the eyes of others. Obscurity makes
a fool of you. It allows people, like Victor in the café, to

imagine all sorts of things: that love falters and weakens when stretched over time and distance; that ignorance surely originates from dislike and has its roots in a family row or some significant inadequacy on your part. Being in obscurity marks you out as a failure. It allows otherwise kindly people to say to you when your sister dies, 'Well, it wasn't as if you really knew her.' It makes you fair game for all the crass insensitivity that's out there, founded as it is upon the mistaken supposition that those you do not see you cannot grieve.

That's why Victor had such a big problem with the degree of remoteness – and perhaps imagined familial hostility – that my lack of a photograph implied. A family photograph is proof of a relationship. Without a photograph there is no case for a relationship, no basis upon which a stranger may be persuaded that the sister you are seeking, post-mortem, is one you cared about and vice versa. Sure, Victor was a bully, but his implication that without a recent photograph you cannot be a proper sister was not unrelated to the assumption made by a significant number of our friends that her death must have been some sort of relief to the family.

There was something symbolic about no photograph. There was something about its non-existence that suggested I might be misguided to claim that Catherine was still mine in some incontrovertible way, and I hers. There was something about its non-existence that gave credence to the belief already held by some outside the family that our relationship with Catherine was sufficiently lacking that our grief must surely be unsustainable. I know there are people who believe that her illness caused us embarrassment, who thought her death no more than a sorry conclusion to a sorry, wasted existence. I know they believe that hers was a life best put down quietly, her memory to be disposed of without fanfare or at least confined to a very small space in our hearts. I know they think these things and I know they are wrong. They are not bad people but collectively they lack sympathy and insight. Some do not understand. Others do not take the trouble to imagine. Some perhaps cannot bear to.

I found myself in that Bristol café, as I did so often in other times and other places, with no evidence to support my search for my sister. I had nothing with which to prove myself to Victor or anyone else. I had precious little information and hardly any working knowledge of Catherine's life. I had never, for example, been able to account for her time. Had I looked at the clock at mid-day or seven in the evening, I would not have been able to imagine what she was doing. I had no notion of when she might be getting up, making toast, sitting in an armchair, painting or listening to music. For some years I had an Australian boyfriend and when he and I were apart, which was quite a lot, we could account for one another's time. It wasn't complicated. For the best part of each of our days the other one of us was asleep. The relationship was very cheerful so the accounting was relaxed, but it made a difference. It reduced the gap between us.

Accounting for another's time is a big deal, particularly if you can't do it. I knew Catherine but I did not know about her because I had no details. I didn't know where she went, whom she knew or what she liked to do. I had no picture of her daily life. I wasn't sure if she had any friends. I never imagined her as a picture of physical health but I was unaware that she had cancer. Worst of all, by the time she was already dead I would never have guessed that she wasn't still in her flat, alive.

And yet what if I'd had all the details? Details do not amount to knowledge because a lot of details are only information. Real knowledge of another person is dependent upon mutual understanding. But does understanding of a family member, or at least the capacity for it, lie in awareness of domestic specifics or is it writ in blood? You can know how your sister pulls on a jacket or rolls a cigarette or picks up a paintbrush, but it doesn't mean you understand her. Siblings can have the same parents and grow up in the same house, with the same family jokes, the same knives and forks, even the same-sounding laugh, but that doesn't guarantee a profound comprehension of one another, only familiarity. Consanguinity is perplexing for it promises so much yet ensures nothing. It is perfectly possible to find that in adult life your sister is little more to you than a recognisable feature of your own extended landscape.

Try telling that to the Victors of this world. I could have shown him a photo and it would have fallen into place for him. He would have seen that while Catherine looked androgynous, and I feminine, she and I had the same-shaped face. He would probably have realised that if she'd eaten enough and not smoked her body into submission, our similar build might have been fleshed out in comparative, recognisable ways. He might have been able even to accept, however strange, that Catherine/Steve with her crew cut and man's jacket resembled this woman before him with her long hair and lipstick. He would have had evidence of familiarity and would almost certainly have taken it for a degree of intimacy. He understood that my asking him about my sister was weird because to disclose that degree of ignorance to a stranger is tantamount to an admission of deficiency. It is like divulging that you have been derelict in your duty as a family member and are therefore a pretty shoddy person.

However, should you confess the tiniest detail about another person you will, if it's the right sort of detail, confer instant status upon yourself. Women know this only too well, and for some it is a social skill at which they excel. If, for example, one woman tells another with *faux* nonchalance that a man they both like can't stand being tickled but loves Marmite on toast for breakfast, she is laying claim to him. The first detail implies physical intimacy, the second an overnight stay, the two together, bed. But what counts is the sum total of the details. They add up to both a warning and a statement: he's mine. Likewise, if a mother tells someone who is trying to curry favour with her by producing sweets for her children that they don't like Smarties, she is in effect telling that person to get lost. She is also doubling the insult by lying (no small child rejects Smarties) but she knows that as the mother of young children her status is as good as inviolable. This means that she can produce almost any detail she likes in order to assert her position, however spurious that detail may be.

The shorthand provided by the use of personal information is extremely valuable currency and while most women know implicitly how to use it to their advantage when sexual or maternal territory is being asserted and there is some perceived risk of conflict, shorthand matters in every relationship. And it is not the details alone that count, it is how they are used and what they reveal about your status and your responsibilities. Your status and responsibilities as a sister are much less clearly defined than your status as a mother or wife. Nevertheless, they are broadly understood to include a wide range of personal contact with your sibling as well as some knowledge of her day-to-day physical and emotional life.

The social expectations built into the role may not be great but they are certainly sufficient to make it clear to an outsider when you do not meet them. If I'd visited my sister regularly and taken to her in person the gifts that instead I sent through the post, our relationship would make more sense to a lot of people. If I could tell them that the family had rallied when she was ill and gathered around her bedside as she lay dying, our grief would be more explicable. To put it brutally, it would be worth more. But grief is regarded as a fairly reliable measure of your connection to someone, and so presumably you get what you deserve, which in our case was essentially a message after someone's death that they had left without saying goodbye. If you haven't put sufficient time into the relationship, or so the thinking goes, then you do not fully deserve your grief because you haven't really earned it.

'I'd have visited her, definitely,' was said to me more than once after Catherine died. 'I'd have just turned up.' Well, the last family members who did that, and with the best of intentions, had the door firmly shut in their faces. They knew it was a risk. We all knew what a bad idea a surprise visit could be. None of the family doubted Catherine when she wrote and telephoned but insisted that she could not handle face-to-face encounters. None of us thought she was anything but serious. Each of us respected her wish to be left alone, to make the running in the relationships that we had with her. Quite apart from which, if an adult wants to live in a particular way, then who is another adult to dispute that, family member or not? Shared genes do not come with a bill of rights.

As for me, I was motivated almost as much by fear as respect. That fear was of the sister who had been violent when younger, who had threatened to kill me in our parents' orchard with a long-bladed sheath knife when I was six years old. She apologised profusely when I broke down in tears, begging. She pulled me awkwardly into her hip and told me she hadn't meant it, but the damage was done. After that episode I was frightened of being alone with Catherine. I was unnerved by her extremes, by her manic muttering, grinning, swearing and laughter. The laughter was the worst: it was specific in character, seeming always to imply the private enjoyment of a sinister joke, a joke which might well be at your expense. I was alarmed by the grotesque and freakish tales of conspiracy and threat that she spun when she was at her most psychotic. It occurs to me now that as a child I was frightened of Catherine in exactly the same way that I was terrified of ghosts or witches. When exposed to the voluminous extravagance of her terrifying and fanatical psychosis I believed in her demonic capabilities as fervently as I believed in the supernatural.

Which meant that all those years later I was scared that if ever I entered her home she might stab me after all, as if time had stopped and we were suspended in a moment that could only be resolved one way. I had a permanent and unpleasant fantasy of being trapped in a gloomy hallway, Catherine with her back against the front door, a knife in her hands, grinning. I imagined trying to talk sense into her and failing. Throughout my twenties, whenever I half-considered an impromptu dash westwards towards her, I was prevented by the thought that she didn't want a visit from me or anyone else. Turning up unexpectedly would only make her angry, which wasn't fair on her, but I believed it was also dangerous. If angry, she might feel cornered and attack me. I worried that if I arrived at her flat bearing home-made stew and a bunch of flowers I would be found dead later, in a stew of my own blood.

I know now how very unlikely that would have been. I have learnt how peaceable my sister was in her later years and rather than compounding my regret at not having seen her, knowing that has eased it. She was happier in her forties, clearly, than she had ever been in her teens and twenties. The aggression had dulled, the mood swings were more muted and less flamboyant. Her illness had burnt itself out to a certain extent although it was still the cloak in which her personality was very tightly wrapped. But she had built a life for herself. She had a routine, had found friends in George and Jo and Richard McKay, and allies in the local community. She knew where to find company, a free lunch, and the right quantity of conversation without intervention or involvement. All this was something for which to give thanks.

So I don't explain to the people who thought I failed her that it isn't easy to respect someone's wishes to be left alone but it is right. I don't tell them that when a schizophrenic says they cannot see you because it is too painful, they mean it. I don't explain that when Catherine made this clear it was not a personal rejection of me but of the assumed requirements of our mutual relationship, most of which she could not meet or respond to. I don't tell them that I would have loved to have been a more fully functioning sister to Catherine; that I would have loved us to share Chinese take-aways and rented movies, loved us to go for walks together. I do not explain myself because few people seem to believe that such simple things were genuinely impossible. After I married but before I had children I felt confident enough in Catherine, and in my husband's ability to protect us, to invite her to my home. She wasn't capable of making the internal journey necessary for the trip, let alone the physical one, but she knew the invitation was sincere. Of course, it would have been nice if she could have made it. It would have been nice if she hadn't been ill.

But ill she was and whether her illness caused her need for such a strong degree of seclusion, or greatly compounded an existing need, no one can be sure. What I am sure of is that I lost Catherine before I had a chance fully to understand what it was I had lost. I was only nine by the time she made her most decisive exit from our family life together. By that time, she was twenty-two and had been repeatedly sectioned in more than one psychiatric hospital. She had been to India and back, twice, and returned to England to a cycle of parental home, bedsits, jobs she couldn't keep, more hospitals and two brief, pointless spells in prison, for threatening behaviour and petty thieving. After that, she followed her boyfriend to Bristol. He didn't last and was replaced by a puppy that didn't last either. No one could quite bring themselves to ask what had happened to it but it was probably given away, like many things in Catherine's possession. She phoned and wrote home frequently, usually with requests for money, and there were visits to her in Bristol, but I was fifteen when she next came home. Her bedroom there contained old toys and Tibetan clothes and prayer beads but it no longer smelt of tobacco. Of the different types of music in the house, none was hers. Perhaps this wasn't surprising. She was twenty-eight by then, after all. But there was an air of permanence to Catherine's absence that there wasn't when the others left home, a sense that she might never again return, a hunch that was later correctly borne out by events.

When our parents lost her is hard to say. They knew something was wrong from babyhood. They knew that Catherine did not respond as other babies did, recognised that she was more easily distressed and harder to comfort than was to be expected. As a newborn, her cry was unusually high-pitched, something most often associated with babies who have suffered brain damage during birth, which she didn't. When they lost her, finally, it was the ultimate blow in a series of blows that had lasted for forty-seven years, and to which they had grown miserably accustomed. She was born very hard to reach, began to go missing almost as soon as she arrived.

Our parents have said that her death was not the shock it might have been had she been one of the rest of us. The phone call out of the blue from an unknown official had always been a strong possibility as far as they were concerned. Dead in her flat for two weeks, police breaking the door down. Dead in the street, exposure. Murdered. Overdosed on drugs perhaps. Possibly suicide. For years they had thought it would be worse than it turned out to be, until the reality was actually just as bad because dead is dead and gone is gone, and she was their child, their first daughter. The ultimate blow in a series of blows, Catherine's death marked the beginning of a second, different type of grief for them to endure, and brought with it nothing to mitigate the first.

When Catherine released me from her grip that sunny morning in the orchard, and replaced her sharp knife in its lavishly embroidered sheath, I ran towards the house hysterical. After she had made her protestations of sorrow, and a promise never to hurt me, I had been issued with a warning:

'If you ever tell them what I said, I will kill you. Do you understand? I will kill you.'

I tore upstairs and banged hard on the bathroom door. It was still early, before breakfast. Catherine and I had been down the orchard either to feed the hens or maybe just to go for a walk but it was well before eight o'clock, probably nearer seven.

My father was shaving. My mother was wrapped in a damp towel after a bath. Howling with sorrow and guilt, I betrayed my sister.

'Please don't tell her I told you! Please don't tell her I told you!'

Catherine was not banned from the house. She was never banned from the house despite her sometime attempts to destroy it and her occasional threats to the people inside. But she was considered a danger to me and possibly to others. This much I know was made clear to her. She went away for a while, came back, floated around the place smoking and muttering, but I was no longer left alone with her. She was supervised, an object of worry and suspicion. Catherine was in a sorry state and home is the most obvious place for a sick child to be. Except that she was now a sick young adult, her agitation hovering on the perimeter of violence. In her presence people felt intimidated. She was twitchy and aggressive. She provoked qualms and hesitations. Overseeing her was the only thing to do and the most loving. I bet it didn't feel that way, either to the overseers or to Catherine.

The pain of this imposition upon Catherine's freedom, and the further unravelling of their trust in her, belonged to our parents and no one else. A shadow was cast over her in order that others should remain safe but it covered our parents also. And thus I would not wish to make too much of the situation, at least from my own perspective. Plenty was concealed from me and I don't remember a lot about that time. Or rather, I don't remember the details the way that an adult would, and what I do does not trouble me. It didn't trouble me at the time, either. I felt perfectly secure and happy. I went to school and returned home to biscuits and milk. There were dogs and cats to play with, neighbouring children up the lane. Days began with boiled eggs and ended with bedtime stories. The house was full of people coming and going but I had the self-absorption of all small children. Catherine was an influence but her illness did not impinge upon me as it did upon her and others, especially our parents.

It is true that several memories of her have drama as their key element. The earliest of these was being told she was in hospital for the first time; I can still recall my shock and anguish because I thought she might die. But mostly I remember the good bits. She was fun and she was wild. She sang, and when she took a summer job at a local farm she learned to drive a tractor. She smuggled me in to her bed where I was instructed in Tibetan chants. She drew pictures for me, anything I asked for, quickly and accurately. 'Can you draw my lion, please?' She did. 'Draw the dogs! Draw a dragon! Draw me!' She taught me how to cartwheel. We perfected the double somersault. She would lie on her back and raise her feet. I would place my stomach on her feet and tuck my own legs into the backs of her knees so that we made an imperfect, but effective, circle. It took days of practice to get the roll right but she was patient and precise. 'Draw you and me being in the circus!' In her room we were singers and artists, on the lawn, acrobats. At night she gave me chewing gum, Wrigley's Spearmint, which was strictly forbidden to me at any time. She was daring and anarchic, and anarchy appeals to children as long as they know it is safe. Mostly it was, or at least it felt that way to me.

I wish she were still alive. I wish she were alive because she was too young to die. I wish she were alive to enjoy the things that brought her joy. I wish she were alive because she wanted to be. And I dearly wish she were alive for my parents because it isn't right for your children to die before you.

I do not wish she were alive for me because there would be something selfish in that. She lived her life for no one else and in dying deprived no one of her care. I still miss her, though. I cannot see her again, can't write to her or talk to her, and I would like to do that. I miss not knowing what might have been. Most of all, I wish I had known years ago what I know about her now. I won't have to worry about her when I'm old, as that friend so helpfully pointed out. Well, I should have liked the option.

I think about the sister I loved as a child. I think about the altered love I felt for her adult self, a love that had less and less to go on and therefore required more conscious effort. Over the years, there were fewer building blocks available for any kind of significant relationship and her absence had a numbing effect. So when I think about her now there is sadness but no pretence. I do not pretend that her loss left the same kind of void in my life that the death of someone closer would have done. I would not insult our relationship by claiming that it was something it was not. I did not love her as I love my other siblings, do not mourn her death as I know I would mourn any of theirs. I do not miss her as a component part of my daily life because she was not. But she was built into me, a portion of my internal mechanism. When she died, my insides were not ripped asunder but they were partially rearranged. Her passing has left its mark.

Schizophrenia locked Catherine in and it locked us out. She was the only kind of sister to me that she was capable of being, and I was the only kind of sister to her that it was possible to be, given the circumstances. I wasn't very much of a sister in the end but there wasn't a lot of room in which to manoeuvre, and while I still think sometimes of all the things I might have done, I could have been worse. I could have pestered or forsaken her. I did not do either. I lived where her illness dictated, on the very fringes of her life, where my childish adoration mellowed to adult concern and bewilderment fed upon a surplus of ignorance. I lived a long way from Catherine, my bountiful life a far cry from hers, but I never got out from under the umbrella of her illness. I was unfamiliar, unaware and uninformed but not, I hope, unkind.

The Remains of That Day

I didn't go straight home from Bristol that night. I sat on the train, my mind awash with George and Victor and the Methodist Centre, and stayed on it all the way to London. My friend, James, was having a launch party for his first novel, and because James is a film-maker, the party was in Soho, in a street full of film studios and editing suites. The venue was a classic Soho affair; small, crowded, loud, trendy, and on this midsummer evening, steamy and humid.

When I arrived, the party was gathering momentum, with James at its centre standing tall, looking hot and jovial. I squeezed my way through the crush of writers and actors in damp linen and sticky silk, kissed him, told him, 'Congratulations.'

Waitresses were offering champagne and enormous strawberries dipped in thick, expensive white chocolate. The food was thematic: James's novel was about chocolate. I asked for a glass of water. I wanted a cup of tea, Earl Grey, weak, with plenty of milk. I wanted to go home.

But I like James a lot, so I stayed. I talked to his family, then for a while to some mutual friends, then to a couple of TV actors.

'Isn't James incredible?' said one.

'He is,' I agreed.

'Yeah, I love James,' said the other.

'Yes,' I said.

'He's a great guy.'

'Yes, he is.'

'A really great guy.'

'Yes.'

'And this book of his is meant to be really good. I haven't actually read it yet.' He held up his copy like a totem. 'But I'm going to.'

'Right,' I said.

'You read it yet?'

'No, not yet. But I've got a copy, too.'

'Yeah,' said the first actor, 'Ah well, good on him. I couldn't write a book, not if you paid me.'

I said, 'They did pay him.'

'Yeah, but you know what I mean. I just really admire writers. You know, writers are just amazing.'

'Well, I wouldn't say that, necessarily,' I countered. 'They're no more amazing than anyone else.'

'You're a writer, aren't you?' he asked.

'Yes.'

He grinned cheerfully and raised his glass.

'There you are, you see. Amazing! You know, you just sit at home, waiting for inspiration.'

I said, 'It's not actually like that. If you waited for inspiration, you'd never get anything written. You just work normal hours.'

'Yeah, but don't you have to be, like, really self-disciplined to write a book?'

'Yes.'

He pointed his finger triumphantly.

'There you are, you see. Self-discipline. Amazing. I couldn't do that.'

A publisher I knew, but whose name escaped me in the heat, made her way to me.

'My God, I haven't seen you in ages! How are you? What are you working on right now?'

I told her I was just at home with the baby and I made it sound as boring as possible so that she'd lose interest in me. It worked a treat. I began to edge my way towards the door and the relative cool of the street on to which the party had now overflowed. I was nearing success until I bumped into another woman I knew.

'Hello stranger, what are you up to?'

I adopted the same tactic. It failed. She was having IVF. Desperate for children, she wanted to know everything there was to know about motherhood.

'So is it just the most incredible thing?'

I said it was but I didn't bang on about it. I didn't want to make her feel bad.

But she wanted to know. She wanted to know all about my daughter; what she ate, whether she was walking, who she looked like. And she couldn't stop smiling at me, either, which was unnerving.

I did my best but all I could think about was George and the sandwich that he made every morning for my sister.

'Is teething hell?' she asked.

'I don't really believe in teething.'

'What do you mean?'

'I think it's an excuse for every last mood that a baby has. Babies are people. People are moody. People get tired or uncomfortable or fed up.' I could hear the impatience in my voice and felt badly about it. 'But mothers want reasons for the moods and teeth are easy. I'm not saying teething is a total myth but I think it's mostly a myth.'

'But what about when the teeth are actually coming through?'

'Well, that can take months.'

'Oh.' She looked at me quizzically. 'So I don't have to worry about teething, then?'

'I wouldn't if I were you. There are worse things.'

'What about colic?'

I thought about Catherine's teeth, which were stained yellowy-brown from cigarettes even in her teens, and wondered when she had last been to a dentist. I remembered vaguely that in one of her letters to me she had complained of terrible toothache. I think she said she'd had to have the tooth out in the end. And George had mentioned her buying Nurofen for toothache.

'How do you cope with that?'

'Sorry?'

'Colic. How do you cope with that?'

The heat was making me less and less charitable.

'I haven't really had to.'

I deeply regretted my tone. I didn't mean to sound hostile. I just so badly wanted to be at home, not making small talk at a London party. I wanted to shut out James's nice friends who were only trying to be friendly. I wanted to put away the day, with all that it contained and all that it had revealed to me, and not think about it again for a long, long time. I wanted to bury it. Suddenly, I remembered a beggar child in Calcutta whom I used to pass by regularly when I was there. He buried himself. Each morning, he would place his head in a deep hole in the pavement, and keep it submerged all day, earning tossed coins from impressed foreigners. He became famous for it eventually, his photograph appeared in a Sunday newspaper and was syndicated around the world. 'Head in the sand, Calcutta-style,' one newspaper wrote. I don't think I ever tossed him any coins. I remember being too bewildered by every aspect of the spectacle, including my own witness.

'You're lucky,' said the woman, earnestly. 'My friend's baby, he's had it since he was born and he's eighteen months now. They've tried everything. I've told them they've got to try acupuncture. I mean, I don't know if you can have it for children but it's worth finding out.'

I said nothing.

'Have you tried acupuncture?'

'I haven't.'

'Oh, you should, it's fantastic. I swear by it. And my friend, she's just started having it, her daughters are five and three now, and she says she wishes she'd had it years ago.'

I was beginning to feel really desperate. I didn't want to be rude to this woman but I felt possessed by a horrible combination of lethargy and panic. It was the wrong place and the wrong time. I made my excuses, wished her luck, said goodbye to James, and squeezed out as fast as I could.

The younger of the two actors was in the street, champagne glass in hand.

'Going already?' he asked. 'The night is young.'

I smiled.

'Baby at home. The nine fifteen train. All that.'

He winked.

'Got ya! Another time, maybe.'

I began to walk towards Regent Street. The people who passed me were vivacious and purposeful. They had places to go, intentions. A young woman knocked into me by mistake, giggling as she fed her boyfriend a bite of her apple. Her body formed a pleasing curve as she leaned into his. They were beautifully abandoned, there on the street, and it occurred to me that although I knew exactly how that felt, I couldn't remember.

A middle-aged man stepped out of a restaurant into my path. He smelt freshly showered, full of possibility. I wondered when I would again feel part of everything around me or whether that was it, now; whether the creeping effect of Catherine's death had disconnected me permanently from the mains of life. I felt fused. I was ready to cry but only inwardly. It is a peculiar feeling. My stomach twists and I know because I can feel it that my mouth forms a sour downward turn, but there are no tears. They tend to arrive a few days later, over something meaningless.

My mind raced uncomfortably. I recalled another party, years earlier; a horrible party. I arrived to a room packed with braying urbanites who worked mostly in the media, and I wanted immediately to leave. I turned to do so but became wedged between three men who worked in television and wanted to talk only to each other, about television. Two were so thick in dispute over something that the third man, whose name was Nick, had little choice but to talk to me.

Nick had done a lot of producing and was now consigned to the comfy executive back benches of ITN. He displayed signs of volatility common to the insecure but egregiously vain, and he had the air of a man who had come to expect a lot from his working environment (like company cabs and an elastic expense account) but almost nothing from work itself.

We ambled around a few harmless subjects and then he said, 'What was your surname again?'

'Loudon. That's my maiden name, that I write under.'

'I thought that's what you said. Loudon . . . rings a bell.'

He's read my books, I thought. How nice.

'Loudon,' said Nick. 'There was a doctor called Loudon, in Oxfordshire somewhere.'

I was not expecting that.

'Yes,' I said, 'he's my— '

'Yeah, that's right. He had a daughter who got busted for being in a drugs ring at some posh school. I was working for a newspaper then, it was my first job.' He took a swig of wine. 'I had to sit outside his house for a week, waiting for the family to come out. Poor sods. There were several of us there, drugs were a massive thing then, huge taboo. Not like now.'

I opened my mouth to say something but he continued.

'Christ, I feel a bit bad looking back on it, but it was a nice job for a cub reporter. Out of the office all day. There was a river there, I seem to remember.'

'Strictly speaking,' I managed to say, and my voice sounded disembodied to me, 'it's a large stream, not a river.'

'Oh yeah?' said Nick. 'You know it then? You connected?'

'I am connected,' I said. 'He's my father. She's my sister.'

To his credit, Nick blushed.

'I see.'

I wasn't going to help him. I remembered the stories of the press outside my parents' door.

'She okay now, your sister?' he stumbled. 'Sorted herself out?'

'No,' I said, 'she's not okay.'

'Couldn't kick the habit?' he asked.

'It's not that straightforward.'

'No,' he said, 'it never is, is it.'

There was a pause and then I said, 'I must go. I'm meant to be somewhere else.'

'Sure,' said Nick, with enormous relief. 'You go.'

'Nice to meet you,' I lied. How I wished I could bring myself to say something different, something truthful.

'Mary?' said Nick.

I turned back slightly. Was he pleading with me?

'Yes.'

He looked over my head into the distance somewhere and then he coughed.

'Tell your Dad I'm sorry.'

I've seen Nick since. I've seen him four times, to be precise, at the sorts of parties I have to go to for work sometimes, and each time, I have thought how much worse it must be for him to see me across a room, rather than the other way around.

*   *   *

He wasn't the only one who knew Catherine. After she died, she surfaced quite frequently. At a friend's house, I met a woman who had been at school with her. At a literary festival, I met another who had known her in Oxford.

'I used to be a student counsellor for the university,' she told me. 'We were open every evening, and when she was living in Oxford Catherine would come in to see us regularly. She used to talk to me a lot. I thought she was an incredible person, a really special person.'

She was everywhere, it seemed, this dead sister of mine. In life, people can be located. Even though I had never known the inside of her flat, or her timetable, at least I had known that Catherine was in Bristol. In death, she was dislocated. Now, she was everywhere and yet nowhere at all, most residual of all in her absence.

Some time after James's party, I was sitting at a friend's long kitchen table thinking about a man who would have been around it too, if he hadn't died two days beforehand. I had seen him only a couple of months earlier. He looked ill then but I had no idea how ill. I glanced across at the hostess, my friend, who had made supper for twenty of us. She was young still, my age. Her sister was not long dead. She was much closer to her late sister than I was to mine, and fought hard on her behalf while she was alive. The chances that her sister crossed her mind that day were pretty high.

How many dead were at supper that night? How many parents, siblings, spouses, friends? How many minds were crossed that day by how many heavenly bodies? It was a big party and the guests were not all young. God forbid, were there children there, too?

The woman across the table asked me about my family. She was roughly my age, late thirties. She already had two dead sisters and a dead mother.

I thought, We are the repositories of the dead. We are their only remaining place on earth.

'I'm so sorry,' I said to her. 'That's a lot to cope with.'

She nodded and ran her finger slowly around the top of her glass.

'Not a day goes by,' she replied.

Telegram

10th September 1973

DR LOUDON MILL HOUSE WANTAGE BERKS

PLEASE TELEPHONE 930 232 BETWEEN 10 AND 5.30
ABOUT YOUR DAUGHTER CATHERINE IN INDIA
FCO

Indian Summer, 1973
A Father's Diary

Tuesday September 18th

On the plane, I read that brilliant book by Oliver Sacks called *Awakenings*, about the effects of L-dopa on post-encephalitic Parkinson patients. For reasons it is difficult to put in words it had a particular resonance with the nature of my journey and with the sensation in jet travel of being suspended motionless. One bit hit with a particular force. Sacks says:

> *I kept thinking of something Joyce wrote about his mad daughter: 'Fervently as I desire her cure, I ask myself what will happen when and if she finally withdraws her regard from the lightning-lit reverie of her clairvoyance and turns it upon that battered cabman's face, the world.'*

It was six days that seemed like six weeks and was more of an ordeal than I had ever expected.

Wednesday Sept 19th
Delhi.

Below, an enormous plain with a mosaic of small fields. Vast irregular areas of floods - some encroaching on villages. But for the floods the pattern looked astonishingly neat. Coming out of the plane, hit by a hot humid blast. I thought it came from the jet engines. It didn't. It's part of the landscape. The sweat breaks out.

Mr Campbell from the Commission appeared. He had come to meet me with an official car. I was enormously grateful. He had to rise before six for that. He has arranged for me to borrow a brand new flat in the compound. ('It's rather like Kew Gardens,' he said, which is just right). He has left me to have the most welcome shave and shower I've ever had. Put on my 'Corsica uniform', pale linen trousers and shirt. Felt new. No longer tired.

The High Commission and living quarters, all new and smart, are in a compound reminiscent of a posh, permanent army camp. There are soldiers in tents outside. I asked why. 'Oh, in case of demonstrations.'

On the steps outside the flat I'm in we noticed a few drops of blood. Fresh. 'Rather ominous,' said Campbell with a grin. Homicide, shaving or menorrhagia? The only sign of human activity is two of the staff immaculate in white tennis clothes, playing tennis earnestly.

Christ, it's hot. Mr Campbell calls it chilly. It's about 95 degrees.

Wed Sept 19th, 11 a.m.

In the air-conditioned entrance of the British High Commission awaiting a hired car that is to take me to Dharamsala.

The staff have been outstandingly kind, efficient and helpful. At nine o-clock, a conference with Mr James and Mr Campbell. I tell them the background story. They showed me the letter from the Dalai Lama's office saying Catherine was in need of care, help and attention.

Mr Ian Wells, an Indian and a sweet man, came in. It was he who went, in response to the Dalai Lama's office, and met Catherine. Catherine was clearly disturbed. She said she had a room but refused to tell him where it was. He understands that she had slept out in the open – in pouring rain.

Apparently, everyone really does know her there and it appears they are kindly and sympathetic. In fact, if anyone tries to hunt her out, any of the Tibetans will hide her. It seems she has charmed them. But it also appears she wanders up to the Dalai Lama's monastery at midnight and the police have to be fetched to bring her away - mainly for her own safety. It appears they like her and want to help. From many sources now, no one doubts

1. She is mentally disturbed
2. She is on drugs
3. She ought to be removed for medical care
4. She will be unwilling to leave.

I don't feel hopeful I will succeed.
I would love to sleep and sleep in a cool room.

But I want to get started now. I want most desperately to see her.

The doctor here who has a small hospital in the compound fixed me up with codeine phosphate against diarrhoea – which I forgot to bring – and general advice. I gather that if I want to eat, I eat curry – or curry. Useful advice on fluids – buy Coke or bottled mineral drinks, or tea. Not water.

Car-hire firm an hour late. The staff here have rung three times, each time the car is 'on its way'. An unpropitious start.

In the High Commission compound there is a noticeboard. On it is a huge, coloured chart of snakes surrounded by ridiculous Peter Sellers-type remarks: 'Some snakes are nice. Very good friends of farmers. You must not kill them.' 'The Cobra. Very poisonous. Kills you at instant once. It hiss then it strike.' Bloody marvellous poster for my morale.

Incredible to think that just over 48 hours ago I was starting a Monday morning surgery in Church St, Wantage.

Ian Wells asked shyly if I could, as a favour, try and retrieve his bath towel which he left in Dharamsala when he went in search of Catherine. Only too happy.

Wed

Car turned up at 12.30. We then found the hire firm had subcontracted. The car had a faulty second gear and the driver spoke virtually no English. Angry exchange on the steps of the Embassy. Indian Head of Transport at the High Commission said he had a friend, guaranteed reliable. Would have car by 2.30.

Mr James carted me off to have lunch with him and his wife in beautiful, cool, air-conditioned flat. They were kindness itself. Fed me and insisted on providing water, water biscuits, cheddar cheese and two cans of beer for the journey. Have never met with such kindness.

2.15, car turned up, American, large, and we started. The crowdedness, slumminess and broken down-ness of Delhi unbelievable. Went to driver's home in the slums to collect his bags and set off on ring road round Delhi. Sacred cows all over the place, slums and hovels everywhere. Buses crammed with Indians standing on bumpers. Carts drawn by camels. Dead dogs sprawled across road. Crowds and crowds and crowds. Heat almost unbearable, between 90 and 100 degrees. Twenty minutes along, car broke down. Carburettor float chamber gone. Driver 'very sorry'. Has gone to find telephone to ring his company and get new carburettor.

I am sitting in the back of the car beside the walls of old Delhi very nearly totally exhausted. Traffic, flies, heat, smell. Things getting worse. It's now ten to four and there are 200 miles to do to the overnight stop. I do not share the driver's optimism about getting there. Even wondering if he is going to come back, or leave the car to join the other roadside wrecks – with me in it. Jesus.

After two hours, the driver and two others turned up in another car and started long argument in Hindi. My temper snapped and I yelled, 'Take me back to the British High Commission. I'm not going on tonight.' So back we went at frantic speed. Back at High Commission I said I'd had enough and could they please recommend a hotel with air-conditioning. Jimmy James was overcome and has wangled me an Embassy car with their best driver to take me up to Dharamsala starting 5 a.m. tomorrow. He and Mr Campbell, the young attaché, have staggered me with their concern and kindness. They stayed on late to get every detail arranged.

Thursday 20th

Fair night.
Woke 10 p.m. with nightmare.
Woke midnight with classic left-sided migraine. Took 3 aspirin.
Woke at 4 with violent acid regurgitation. Got up. Sudden diarrhoea. Oh Christ no – not that, just before the journey.

Breakfast on Jimmy and Cath James's water biscuits and one of Dr Hamilton's codeine phos. tablets.

Car arrives before dawn. Driver immaculate in white uniform, happy smile, short, stout, fiftyish. He drives with consummate skill.

Dawn comes soon. The Delhi plain: flat, dirty and dusty. Straight tarmac roads, tree-lined, the roads teeming. Massive lorries coming down from the Punjab with produce, all labelled 'Public carriers' and covered with Kashmir-shawl like decorations. Beat-up cars of all sorts, bicycles, Indians wandering everywhere, or lying or squatting or pissing. Everybody in middle of the road and every driver leaning on his horn continuously. Madly unsafe. About 11 a.m. having passed numerous dead dogs, we come across three squashed bodies, very dead. Overturned lorry and smashed motor bike. Crowd stands watching. One policeman. Each body surrounded by a circle of bricks. 'Punjab lorry drivers very bad. Drink too much.' says my driver. Comforting.

My bowels heave and gripe. Will I have to join the squatting Indians? Stop for petrol. Toilet is brick-built box in corner. Rush to it through pool of water outside. It isn't water, it's urine. There is no can, lavatory or even hole in the ground. You piss and it runs out through the door. This is an Esso station, one S the wrong way round. I add to the urine pool and grip my bowels tight. Take more codeine phos., lots of it. Back in car, off at 60 mph avoiding death by skill of driver. Heat unbearable. Bowels less pressing but nausea mounting.

After 200 miles, stop at the 'best hotel' for lunch, but really for loo. A grim place. Relief at last – at least there is a lavatory bowl. Look at menu with nausea. Was told lamb is safest. Chose lamb chop and chips and Himalayan apple juice. It comes. It is a cutlet, not a chop. Try a bit, only a small bit. Tastes a bit spicy and then, like a delayed action fuse, it explodes and my lips, palate and tongue are on fire. Drink all the apple juice at once to quench it. Eat one mouthful. Nausea returns. Pay for it uneaten and go back to loo. Christ, I feel awful.

Landscape unbroken, flat. Buildings red brick or mud, all look half-finished, none with any appeal, not even squalid appeal. An awful awful hot sticky septic stinking country. Air scented with cedar wood mixed with faeces.

With just over 250 miles done, we suddenly enter foothills with twisty roads. There are 90–100 miles of this. Nausea and tiredness so bad I have moments wondering if I can stand it. Eventually to Dharamsala. Still as hot as ever. Stop at hotel, book in, rush to loo. Cold shower in concrete hole off room. Fifty per cent restored. OK, now I am ready for it. Up to find Catherine.

Road up to McLeodgang only nine kilometres but seems endless, up and winding. Enter cloud at 6000 feet which obscures all mountains. Suddenly and marvellously cool. Houses of logs and steep overhanging roofs. Troops and barracks along all the road – Sikhs, I think. They look ferocious.

McLeodgang. What an incongruous name. Perhaps it's the shower and the cool but I feel I can cope. An hour ago I didn't.

We arrived in McLeodgang at 4 p.m. The village beautifully situated, consists of two rows of houses and a broad street of market stalls. Crowded, mainly Tibetans, some Tibetan monks, some Indians and about twenty or thirty stoned European hippies.

At the top of the street is the main store run by Mr Nowerjee, who speaks good English. He got me a folding seat and went off to see where Catherine was without saying I was there. He came back shortly and showed me some stairs leading up to a room like a very scruffy hotel lounge with two people in it. One was Catherine slumped on a chair smoking hash and looking slightly glazed. I kissed her but she showed no surprise and total indifference to my appearance. I said I'd come to see her and she said, 'Now you've seen me: so what?' I said we were all worried stiff about her and she said. 'I'm OK. Now, goodbye. I don't want to see you.'

I told her I had letters for her and gave them to her. She scrumpled them up and said she would read them later. She got up and I asked if I could come to her room. She said,

'No. Go away! Go away!' She was utterly hostile and cold. I followed her and she ran and disappeared down the corridor, and around a corner. A small crowd of Tibetans was following her and told me she had gone up some stairs. I went up the stairs and found a corridor with a series of small cell-like rooms, all of them squalid. In each was sitting a group of three or four Europeans smoking pot, and in the third room I found Catherine, hiding. She swore at me to go away and I implored her at least to talk to me. One hippy said with an American accent, 'Take it easy.'

Catherine went out into the road and was surrounded by Tibetans, my Indian Driver and the proprietor of the Hotel who had come up with us. They all refused to let her escape me and implored her to talk to me and go away with me. There was infinite kindness and gentleness in the way they handled Catherine, and compassion for me. By this time I was fighting back my tears. When I touched her she shrugged me off violently. She said she would call the police as I was molesting her. She shouted that I used to be her father but now she was 21 and I no longer was.

I asked her if her mother and brothers and sisters meant nothing but she said there was no law that she should talk to me and she wanted me to go away. She addressed the crowd, not me. This went on and on and finally I walked out through the crowd saying it was no good. I said, 'I've had as much as I can take,' and burst into tears. The Indian driver of my car put an arm round my shoulders and we went back to the general store. Mr Nowerjee brought me a fizzy orangeade – and refused payment for it.

Several people suggested the police and getting her forcibly put in the car. I rejected all these.

She had denied mental illness, countered any suggestion that it was the opinion of many who had been in contact with her by saying I did not speak Tibetan so I could not know, and that it was all untrue. She agreed she smoked hash but denied any other drugs. I said we should drive back down to Dharamsala, and then the driver noticed a punctured back tyre, and as we were looking at it, Catherine disappeared. But while the wheel was being changed, some Tibetans ran over and pointed to her walking up a mountain path. I followed, feeling I couldn't leave it there, and was shown by the Tibetans where she had hidden in a small building.

She yelled again and again, 'Go away!', and yelled that I had to learn that in India everyone was enlightened, that I couldn't understand and I was breaking into the 'inner light'. Up till now I had been quiet. I'd been gentle, emotional and pleading. I continued to be but she yelled me down and suddenly I yelled at her to shut up and listen. She did. I said again that it was love that brought me, that after coming this distance the least she could do was talk to me, and I asked her to come down to Dharamsala. She refused, saying she had an important appointment in meditation that night. I said, 'Break it for me.' She refused but ultimately said she would come down to Dharamsala between 9.30 and 10 tomorrow but if she was not there by 10 she wouldn't come at all and I wouldn't be able to find her.

I don't think she will come. I returned to Dharamsala in despair. I have failed.

An hour later, I met the Superintendent of Police at the social club. At a card table six smartly dressed Indians were playing cards. The Superintendent was tall, thirtyish, good looking, smart tweed jacket, white shirt, tie and grey flannels.

He agreed that she could not be arrested as she had committed no crime. She simply causes embarrassment when she has a spell of nuttiness and appears stark naked or wanders all night. He knows she is sometimes mentally deranged and clearly wanted me to take her away. He suggested forcing her into the car. I turned this down flat. It would confirm her utter hostility to family and there would be no way to prevent her escape on the way to Delhi, or at Delhi, or off the aircraft on the way home. I cannot be her jailer.

He thought the time would come when she would have to be certified and deported by police to Delhi. I said I thought that if it came to that, it was the preferable way.

I returned to the Hotel. I haven't eaten all day and don't want to. Thumping headache but no more diarrhoea thank God.

I feel utterly drained of feeling and emotion. All I want is to get back from this terrible country as quickly as possible. Catherine may survive this or may not. I doubt if we can help. I'm sure I can't.

Friday Sept 21st

Slept reasonably well and woke feeling stronger. Cold shower cold shave. It is cloudless and not too hot (about 70). The air is crystal clear and the view immense. There is no denying that the beauty is breathtaking. To the south are rolling foothills and endless plain and immediately behind Dharamsala are the towering mountains, the Himalayas. The lower slopes are dotted with houses, temples and fields.

Breakfast is edible though far from clean. The tea is good. My driver re-appears for his breakfast. He consented to share my room last night. He really is a sweet man, comes from Pakistan. He has an immaculate uniform of white shirt and trousers and peaked cap with High Commission badge. He 'sirs' me all the time, and I have to ride in the back of the car and am not allowed to open the car door myself. He firmly but politely refused my offer of lunch yesterday and lunched off chapatis provided by his wife outside the restaurant. He has brought a sleeping bag and I thought he was going to sleep in the Cortina although I had pressed him to take a room in the hotel at my expense. Then – when I had gone to bed and turned the light out last night – he shyly came in and took the other bed. We chatted in the dark. He was sympathetic. 'Very, very sad time for you. You very sad father I think. I am sorry.' I asked him about his family. He has seven kids ranging from fifteen to four, two boys and five girls. His wife wants another boy. One girl aged twelve has brain damage of some sort – cannot speak or feed herself. He has taken her to every hospital in Delhi, he says. They all say, 'It is just the 'old brain', when the new brain grow, she all right.' It's clearly hopeless. What right have I to be sorry for myself over Catherine?

It is now 8.30 a.m. I wait for Catherine. I must not be angry, gentleness is the only hope. The driver thinks it unlikely the punctured tyre can be mended.

I face the prospect of 350 miles return journey, the first 80 or 90 over rough winding roads and dry river beds, with misgiving. I anticipate getting to Delhi about midnight.

I think that generally the locals here feel I should kidnap Catherine. 'Very good mental hospitals in Delhi. Some of best in world. They give her injections or treatment.' (This is said with fingers pointed at head.) 'She all right and then she go home with father.' They find it hard to understand my disagreement. They seem to have a touching faith in modern medicine (psychiatric), as if it was simple like treating malaria or dysentery. I am *not* going to be cajoled into lying to Catherine and getting her into the car by subterfuge or force. It would do harm not good. I think they will regard me as feeble. I'll have to put up with that. Driver has mended puncture, bless him.

Saturday, 2 a.m.

I was telephoned yesterday – at 10 a.m. – from the upper village and told Catherine was not coming down, and would I please go up.

I went up. A Tibetan came over and gave me her passport. Through an interpreter he said he no longer wanted to look after it and she was not fit to care for it. So I took it.

Then someone said Catherine had gone up to the monastery, half a mile off, so we drove up. No Catherine but I was shown round the temple. Drove back to the village and spotted Catherine on the road. I got out. She walked off. I called. She ignored me. I ran and caught her and made her talk. She was a trace more civil, said she might come back after Christmas. I said, 'OK then, this is good-bye.' She then said the bank was late, could I lend her 100 rupees. I gave her 200.

Back to the hotel to pay the bill, then to the Police Superintendent (as he had requested). We went over the same ground, and almost as an afterthought I produced her passport and said did he want it or should I take it to Delhi? He said Delhi, and then, flicking through its pages, asked when she arrived in India and suddenly said, 'Her visa has run out.' I said I knew nothing of visas.

Then a long argument started between the Super and his staff, the upshot of which was that

1. Catherine would be deported at once
2. Either I could take her or
3. They would arrest her, lock her up and prosecute and deport.

The Super added that it would be inhumane to prosecute, so I said I would take her. Three policemen were summoned after a long deportation order was made out and signed and we went back again up to McLeodgang.

I was told to wait in the entrance to the general store while they went to get her. A youngish Englishman in semi-Tibetan clothes asked if I was Catherine's father. He told me he had been there two years. He also said that British citizens didn't need a visa. I smelt a rat.

Catherine arrived, escorted by a huge tough Sikh police sergeant and the six of us got in the car. Immediately they started saying she was arrested for losing her passport and being sent to Delhi for a new one. I was nudged to hide her passport in the bag I had in my lap.

We returned to police headquarters. The Super had gone but the District Officer was there. I was furious. I said I would not stand for lies. They got angry and said she was to be deported, the order was signed and sent to Delhi and either I took her or they did it the rough way.

What could I do?

I said I'd take her, and they sent a policeman in the car for the first ten miles.

The journey up here was a nightmare. The one back was worse. We left at 2 p.m. C. was facile, exhibitionistic and exhausting, and a bit psychotic. She was restless and kept hanging out of the window: there she would spit repeatedly, then she made noises on a mouth organ or whistled two notes again and again. Once, she produced some hash and said she would show me how to make a joint. I told her not to. She ignored me and I grabbed the lot and threw it out of the window. She chain-smoked cigarettes and once turned on the driver and abused him for coming to fetch her. I yelled at her for that, but the driver, sweet man, took it in good part and chatted to her all the way to Delhi. Her mood was restless, heartless, facile and deliberately provocative. The driver and I were terrified she would jump out or escape. We drove through the night stopping for tea and a meal. I ate nothing. There were numerous hold-ups with accidents and broken down lorries. Driving was hazardous in the extreme with unlit cyclists, bullock carts, road diversions and no rear lights on many cars.

I felt ominously awake and un-tired, trying to work out how I could control her in Delhi.

Arrived in Delhi at 1.30 a.m. Immediately C. started to create a scene. No she wouldn't share a room, so I was offered a suite of two rooms. She came up and said it must have flowers for meditation, and then said it wasn't fit for meditation (it's an enormously grand suite). She pushed off. I told the hotel staff to let her go but to leave her bed made up in the hope that she wanted to return, and to place the door open. Had a shower, rang the British High Commission, tried to ring home. Would be a three hour delay getting through, so I cancelled the call.

I don't know where Catherine is.

I want to get out of this bloody country.

It's now 3 a.m. No sign of C. She has not come up to bed.

Saturday 22nd, 6 a.m.

Slept solidly for three hours. No sign of Catherine. She hasn't been into the adjoining room of the suite. No appetite. Breakfast = tea and a decaying banana. Went downstairs to hotel entrance. No sign and she hasn't been seen.

Rang Brit High Commission and left message that Catherine had disappeared but I had taken no action yet. The police are called.

The infuriating thing is that I have been made unwillingly to act as C's gaoler and I am sure she believes the attempted deportation was at my instigation and would never believe otherwise. As I thought it would, this has made matters worse for Catherine, not better – and much worse for me, which matters less.

When I get to the British High Commission I feel sick, anxious and weak. They are so sympathetic and helpful I am over-come. These two men and that magnificent driver have saved my reason.

Took a taxi to Pan-Am and booked a flight to Heathrow leaving here at 4 a.m. tomorrow. Outside the temp is 98 and the humidity high. It's like the breath of a feverish patient.

Back to the air-conditioning of the hotel and up to my suite where I booked a call an hour ago to Wantage. Outside, a huge thunderstorm is building up. It has poured with rain. I await telephone call, unable to stir.

Eat the last two of dear Mr and Mrs James's water biscuits – it is 3.30 here and apart from the decayed banana at 7 a.m. it is all I've had. Don't want much more. Not risking another bloody lamb cutlet. Write, snooze, read, wait for telephone. Police in jeeps are searching the bus station and hippy areas for Catherine. Christ what a thought.

Oh Catherine. I had sympathy for your wanting to live up at McLeodgang. The place is so beautiful and you never minded a bit of scruffy squalor. I could even see the attraction of Buddhism perhaps, and most certainly, from a brief look, the kindly gentle appearance of the Tibetans. The hippies were horrible – pale, ill, hang-dog, unhappy, egocentric with a touch of decayed arrogance about them. The Indians hate and despise them but say the Indian Government tolerates them purely for foreign currency. I doubt it, because it can't be much. I suspect the Indian Gov. does nothing because it couldn't even organise a dog-fight. Catherine, if you'd been gentle and kind and welcoming I would have done all I could to help you to stay. But it's daft of me to think that. If you'd been well, you would have been welcoming and happy, and you're not well. You're ill. Now where the hell are you? The ache of caring for you comes back quicker than I thought. It will come back worse on the way home. I must expect that, and to expect pain and recognise it for what it is goes a long way to coping with it. Some people have only one child who gets ill, and that must be agony. Thank God for the other children I have. I can't wait to get home.

I don't think I will ever, ever want to see India again. It's the first foreign country I've actually hated.

At two hour intervals I call the operator to see if there is a line to England. Each time they say, 'Very sorry, Government use all lines. Delay two to three hours.' I started trying to phone at 12 and it's now ten to six. This time I blew up, went all Sahib and pulled rank saying I was from British High Commission and it was a very important call. Operator says, 'Very well, I will request then.' We will see. I am stuck here.

Order more coffee.

The sun has come out and the air-conditioning which broke down has re-started. The setting sun shows the domes and buildings of Delhi (I am on the fourth floor with a French window) in an almost favourable light. Delhi is twenty-five miles across and every inch swarming.

Still ten hours before the 'plane leaves. No one has rung to say C. has been found. I was asked if I thought she was a suicide risk. I replied that I had been in medicine long enough to avoid a dogmatic answer but I really thought not.

7 p.m. Jimmy James rang me from his home to ask if there was anything more he could do. He really is pure gold.

7.15. Operator rang to say telephone lines from Bombay out of order.

8.00 p.m. There has been a power cut since 7.20. Internal telephone works and I ring for candles with anger about life mounting.

9.45 p.m. Still can't sleep.

Sunday 23rd, 3 a.m.

Delhi airport.
No news of C. being found. I half expect a posse of police to arrive with her in tow. But they won't.

9 a.m., on the plane. I must have suddenly gone to sleep at take-off because I know we landed at Karachi for an hour and have only a vague recollection of being shaken and shaken by an air hostess to put the seat forward for the landing.

Once awake it's impossible not to think of C. and of what else I might have done. I had set myself with determination to be quiet and gentle. More than once I was within a hair's breadth of real fury. I had no end of advice – discipline, deportation, certification, love, affection, even 'You a doctor: can't you put something in her tea?' – and the advice came from policemen, storekeepers, the hotel owner, Mr Mahomed the kind driver, Tibetans and monks. All desperately well meant.

When I say now that I honestly don't think it would have made any difference I don't know whether it is honesty or self-justi-fication. My tendency for optimism in the past two years, hoping she will recover with treatment, now appears to be cowardice on my part. She is very ill. Perhaps I should have had her arrested in Delhi as soon as we got there (even although I suspected the deportation order was bogus) and then certified. The trouble is I just don't know how mad she is. Though she is very close to it, I am not sure she would be certifiable at home, so if one got her home by brute force she would disappear – probably at once, and probably to people less gentle than Tibetans.

The thoughts, the guilts and the shame of failure just goes round and round.

Out of the window is an airstrip in the desert but otherwise it is unchanged for more than half an hour – that's about 250-300 miles. It's vast.

I was right in forecasting that the pain would return on the way home. A bit worse than I thought. Out of the window, one and a half hours solid of desert at over 500 mph.

Lost and Found

Catherine had been there all along at the hotel in Delhi. As soon as our father arrived in England he phoned for news of her, expecting none.

She had spent the night hiding in the bushes in the hotel garden. She was still there in the morning, laughing, when one of the staff members came across her. He said she seemed quite happy to be found. He said she seemed to think it was funny.

One hot summer night, almost a year later, the rest of the family arrived home from a holiday in Corsica.

Every window in the house was lit up. Smoke curled from the left-hand chimney. The front door was open.

Music was coming from the sitting room, or rather, music was being played in the sitting room, on a recorder. A pennywhistle my mother would have called it. The sound it made was thin and solitary.

My father walked into the room. We all followed.

Catherine was sitting cross-legged in front of a blazing fire, one of the dogs snuggled against her with its nose in her lap.

'Puss!' my father cried out, using the name my parents called her at home.

'Oh, Puss.'

'Hi,' said Catherine, beaming up at us all. 'I thought I'd come home.'

*　　*　　*

Then it began: the terrible cycle of bedsits, prisons, and psychiatric hospitals, where I can remember visiting her, pale and mute in a white nightdress and metal bed. I had never seen anyone looking so empty.

The first of these cycles was in Oxford, the second in London, and somewhere along the line, Catherine acquired a boyfriend.

He lived in Bristol, so they went there together, to set up home.

The relationship with him did not last but the one with Bristol did. It was to become the most constant presence in Catherine's life, the place where she would valiantly build her adult future upon the ruins of a tormented youth.

This Other Outlaw

On an occasional table before me was a plate with four
ginger biscuits and two warm, fresh scones. There were
several chairs in the room, none of them matching, a picture
of wild flowers, a crucifix on a plinth, a stack of magazines
and a small television. There was a gas fire in the fireplace.
I knew from the experience of writing my first book, which
took me to visit a lot of modern convents, that this was
about as typical a sitting-room for contemporary nuns as
you could find. As such, it felt familiar to me. On the wall
was a stitched sampler. It read: *Love is always ready, To
Excuse, To Trust, To Hope.*

Three nuns lived here, including Sister Paul. The other two
were out. Sister Paul was in the kitchen, making a pot of
tea. It was she who had returned my call to the Sisters of
Saint Joseph. It was Sister Paul, and not a Sister Margaret,
who had known my sister. Of course, Catherine's Sister
Margaret may have existed elsewhere but it was possible that
Steve Shepherd had simply got her name wrong.

I was amazed when she first opened the door to me. Her
voice and manner on the phone had led me to expect a much
younger woman.

I remarked upon it, when she returned with the tea tray.

'You've got such a young voice on the phone.'

'Everyone says that. I'm eighty-one.'

'You sound about forty. Don't look much over that, either.'

Sister Paul beamed with pleasure but it was not flattery

on my part. She possessed an openness of character that translated, as it does in a few people, into a spectacular freshness of feature.

'Not that forty is any better than eighty-one,' I said, keen that she should not mistake me for someone who believes in the supremacy of youth over the majesty of octogenarian vigour. 'On the contrary. There was an actress once who said, when congratulated on her sixtieth birthday by a younger woman for not looking sixty, "Honey, this is what sixty looks like."'

'Oh, I like that,' said Sister Paul.

'It's good, isn't it.' I gestured towards her, 'This is what eighty-one looks like.'

'You can come here again,' said Sister Paul.

The house in which she and her fellow Sisters lived was in a fairly grim part of the city, an area that was dull rather than appalling, containing nothing that I could see to lift the spirits but plenty to diminish them. Terrace after terrace of dark brick and stuccoed Victorian houses. Busy roads circumnavigating dead roads, residential streets with a lot of parked cars but no one around. No green spaces. No light in the middle of the streets.

The room in which we were sitting with our tea and scones was bow-windowed. The light was on but it was still naturally dark. I have often thought that the Victorians suffered from a sort of collective depression when it came to architecture. So much of what they created – whether on a grand or modest scale – inspires gloom, at least in me.

'And I don't care how wonderful people say the Victorians were,' grumbled my friend Sue once, when she was halfway through renovating her own Victorian terraced house, with steadily increasing disrespect for their inattention to right angles and their botched plasterwork, 'they were shite builders.'

'Your sister, you know,' said Sister Paul. 'She had great self-respect.'

'She did?'

'Oh aye.' She nodded fervently, her Scots intonation evident. 'She was always so clean. She carried herself well. She kept herself nice. And her face always lit up when she smiled.'

I thought, All round, that's not a bad epitaph.

'You can be very proud of her,' said Sister Paul, 'I think she was a lovely person. Do you take milk?'

'Yes, please.'

'Sugar?'

'No, thank you.'

Sister Paul poured some tea for herself. I asked her which part of Scotland she was from.

'From Glasgow. Do you know it?'

'Not well. I went there for a weekend once with a boyfriend, that's all. It's a handsome city.'

'Oh, it's a lovely city, yes,' Sister Paul rhapsodised, 'a beautiful city, and I owe it an awful lot. I had a wonderful education in Scotland, free, because we couldn't have afforded it at the time. Now, have you,' asked Sister Paul, 'brought a picture of your baby?'

'Is the Pope Catholic?'

Sister Paul laughed. I produced a photograph from my wallet.

'Oh, isn't that lovely!' she said. 'Isn't she a sweetie.'

'Well, we think so.'

'And I bet Cathy would have idolised her.'

'She might have. She idolised me when I was a baby.'

'Did she? I could believe that. Ah Cathy, I'm so glad I knew her. I wish I'd known more.'

'I think we all wish we'd known more.'

Sister Paul handed back the photograph of Clare.

'When did you first meet Catherine?' I asked.

'Oh, must have been about two to three years ago. I'd meet her mostly in Stapleton Road. You don't know it, do you, I'll perhaps show it to you when we're going out. But the strange thing is, the last time I saw her, I was crossing over the road and I tried to get her attention but she seemed very preoccupied, which was most unusual. And then I was away visiting my sister in Australia, and when I came back I didn't see her for a bit. I did wonder where she was.

'It was only when Father McKay mentioned your phone call that I heard she was dead. He told all of us. We were a group who had just had a service and he said, "Do any of you know . . .?" and he described her. And we were all people that knew her, maybe only to say a few words, but we were all her friends, every one of us.'

Sister Paul proffered the plate of scones and biscuits.

'My first meeting with her,' she continued, smiling approvingly as I took a scone, 'was when she was going into the church one morning and she greeted me. She didn't know me at the time but she said, "I always go in to light a candle." I said, "That's nice." After that, I often saw her there.'

'Did you see her a lot in the street?'

'Nearly every morning. She'd lope along the road. Do you know her stride?'

Catherine's walk. Another thing I can neither remember nor describe, though it was clearly so distinctive. I recalled Richard McKay's description of it.

'No.'

'Well, she would come along like this,' Sister Paul sprang from her chair, hunched up her shoulders slightly, and limped across the room, 'but as soon as she recognised you, a smile came out instantly and it was like a ray of sunshine.'

I thought how different was this description from some of my memories. It's not that I don't remember Catherine smiling because I do, but my predominant experience of my sister would not bear the same description as Sister Paul's. I'd never heard anyone describe her as so immediately responsive and so consistent. It was nice to hear but it wasn't something that I recognised.

Sister Paul sat down again.

'That's how I remember her,' she was saying. 'And if she'd see me hurrying to Mass in the mornings, she'd say, "You'll be late! You'll be late!"' Sister Paul laughed roundly. 'She had a real sense of humour.'

That I do remember. However, I always used to think of it as dark and strange, not the stuff of easy, everyday exchange. Catherine was witty rather than congenial, sharp ripostes much more her style than gentle banter or back-slapping *bonhomie*. Yet if I recall the jokes and anecdotes in some of her later letters to me I can see that they were fairly prosaic. I realise now that while the familiar spikiness was evident still, her humour had a straightforwardness I failed to perceive at the time because I couldn't see beyond what I remembered of the Catherine of my early childhood. In that instance as in others, powerful memories served as an obstacle to simple observation.

'And as I said before,' Sister Paul continued, 'I never saw her other than clean and tidy, which is wonderful, because in her condition she could have sunk down, you know.'

She frowned and shook her head slightly. 'But where she lived, I don't know. Do you know?'

'Yes,' I replied. 'She lived in the St Phillips area. There are some flats there for people with various mental health problems, and they're assured tenancies, so she could have had it all her life.'

'Did you have to go and clear it?'

I was taken aback by the question, not so much by its directness nor even by how inadvertently close to the bone it was, but by how best it might be answered.

'Well,' I began, 'it wasn't possible to clear it because there was too much stuff, although we did go and take some things. The trouble was, I don't think she'd thrown anything away for some years. I don't mean rubbish, there was just a lot of stuff.'

Sister Paul nodded.

'Stuff that she collected?' she asked.

'Yes.'

'Well,' said Sister Paul, 'that was her little kingdom, wasn't it.'

'I guess it was.'

'And of course there was somebody, a warden in the place, was there?'

'There was a caretaker. A nice man.'

Sister Paul was silent for a moment.

'Strange she should come up all that way, right up to the other end of Stapleton Road and across Eastern Way.'

'Why strange?'

'Because it's a long way. It would have taken her a long time.'

But time was the one thing Catherine had in abundance. I pictured her walking the streets, day in, day out: thanks to Sister Paul's demonstration, she was now slightly hunched, lopsided.

'She had a lot of time,' I said. 'And I expect, from what you've said, and what somebody else has said, that she walked the same route every day.'

'That's right. It seems to me that she did because I never met her on the other side of the road. Never.'

'I don't think she deviated much from her routine.'

'No,' Sister Paul agreed, 'and she kept herself to herself. Did she speak to the Warden at all, do you know?'

'Not much.'

'No,' Sister Paul ruminated, 'she was a very private person, and although she could be nice and friendly with me, it was thus far and no further, you know what I mean? One of the other Sisters here, Sister Bernadette, she told her that she had cancer. I wasn't around at that time, I was in Australia, but when Sister Bernadette stopped seeing her around she never knew she was dead, she just didn't know where she was. We couldn't even ask her where she lived, you see.'

'No. I understand that.'

Sister Paul looked at me with some concern. I think she was trying to impress upon me that Sister Bernadette had not let Catherine down.

'You see that?' She was making sure.

I replied, 'We all know, don't we, that if we pushed her too far—'

'She would retreat.'

'Exactly.'

'And she would not have anything to do with you.'

'No,' I agreed. 'She wouldn't.'

Sister Paul sighed and leaned comfortably back in her chair, scrutinising me gently.

She said, 'It's very hard for you, I think.'

'It's okay.'

'It is?'

I nodded.

'Good.'

She offered me more tea and I accepted. I looked out of the window at the sky. I knew for a fact that the sun shone in Bristol but thus far I had little evidence of my own to support it.

'Ah,' said Sister Paul, 'and you know, she had an impishness about her. Did you ever remember that at all?'

'Oh yes, definitely. But there's a lot I don't. And do you know, it might sound silly but the thing I mind most is that

I don't remember how tall she was. It's odd what you find you care about.'

'How tall?'

'Yes. Was she tall? How tall was she, compared with me?'

'Well, let's see,' said Sister Paul, rising from her chair, 'let me stand up beside you.'

I rose, too, and Sister Paul stood in front of me, looking up into my face. Sister Paul was not tall herself.

'No,' she declared. 'She was smaller than you, she'd be about to your nose.'

'Really?'

I had always had Catherine down as very tall. I guess I never had much opportunity to develop more than a child's-eye view.

'Yes. She was definitely smaller than you.'

Momentarily, I felt slightly dizzy, beside myself somehow. Here I was, asking a woman I had first set eyes upon only that day to confirm my own sister's height. I thought of George, and Richard McKay. What did Catherine eat? Where did she go? How tall was she? That I was dependent upon the kindness of strangers for even the most impersonal of personal details was ever more apparent.

'There was something very strange,' I said, and I told Sister Paul about the vanishing measurements on the kitchen wall.

'They've just gone?'

'Yes. Totally.'

'Now, isn't that strange,' she agreed.

'Isn't it.'

'Was this after she died?'

'Yes,' I replied. 'I think she's removed herself. That's all I can think.'

I remembered it so clearly, that afternoon in my mother's kitchen, asking how tall Catherine was, expecting to find the answer written on the wall.

'I mean, there will probably be a logical explanation,' I said, 'but I don't know what it is. They were there and now they're not. You know, she grew up in the house, she was one of the five of us and there's no reason for her not to be there.'

'Strange. And when was the last time you saw them, do you know?'

'I can't remember.'

Sister Paul said, 'She seems to have separated herself from you, as if she didn't belong.'

I had thought of it slightly differently, simplistically even. I had imagined Catherine removing herself purely because she was dead and no longer existed, temporally at least. That there was no longer any evidence of her growing self on the kitchen wall underlined also the absolute manner of her disappearance from our lives. Her missing initials were consistent with the firmness of her dying self. We were now, in a concrete sense, no longer her 'next of kin'.

'She knew she was different,' said Sister Paul, with confidence.

It all seemed to fit like a jigsaw puzzle for Sister Paul. I wish it did for me.

'That would explain it,' she added, evidently quite at ease with any implication of the paranormal.

I shrugged. 'Maybe.'

'Well, she was different. And I'm certain the Good Lord loved her because I got joy when I met her, you know, I really did. And she enjoyed meeting me too.'

Sister Paul sprang up again, unexpectedly.

'Your sister and I,' she said, 'whenever we met, we'd have all this ceremony.'

She inclined her head and bowed towards me, her hands in a praying position.

'Like this,' she said. 'We'd both do it together. It was lovely.'

'That's how Buddhists greet one another, isn't it?'

'Yes.'

Memories flooded back, of Catherine teaching me that very form of greeting on the sunlit lawn at home; Catherine teaching me Buddhist mantras; Catherine telling me that to greet one another formally and to offer a sign of peace was very important to Buddhists.

'Catherine taught me that when I was little,' I told Sister Paul, 'she and I used to do that.' And I heard my voice squeaking with the excitement of recognition.

'How lovely!' Sister Paul exclaimed, caught up in the moment with me.

I said, 'I don't know if she ever talked to you about it but she was very influenced by Buddhist thinking.'

Sister Paul sat down again.

'That's right. Sister Bernadette said that she used to talk to her about Tibetan monks. I never had that kind of conversation with her. I can only tell you what she and I did, and the fact that it was a joy to meet her, really and truly. But –' Sister Paul broke off for a moment, 'I was very puzzled. I didn't know whether she was a man or a woman, for quite a long time.'

'No. You're not alone in that.'

'Quite a few other people didn't know either.'

'So what did you call her?' I asked. 'What name did you know her by?'

'You didn't. You just didn't. It was just, Good morning. But some of the others knew her as Catherine.'

Sister Paul folded her arms around herself in a gesture of implied self-protection.

'But again,' she continued, 'I think that was also a matter of her holding back from people, her appearing to be mannish. Of course, she dressed in trousers, but I think she was perhaps protecting herself from any male advances.' And she gripped herself with her arms.

'Well, I don't really think she felt comfortable being a woman.'

'No,' said Sister Paul, her hands dropping back into her lap. 'I felt that.'

'And in the last years of her life,' I explained, 'she would often introduce herself as a man, as Steve. She had another name.'

Sister Paul was not surprised.

'Some of her correspondence was to Steve Stevenz,' I explained, 'although her bank account was still in her original name. Richard McKay said that he had to write a letter for her once and when he put some reference to "she" in it, she got very cross with him.'

Sister Paul nodded in agreement.

'She could get angry with you,' she said, 'but only if you infringed or appeared to her to be infringing. And then of course, if you'd any sense, you'd take note and be careful.'

She leaned towards me.

'You know,' she said, her voice serious, 'I had an interesting experience the other day. I believe in having a lot of joy, you know, that laughter is the best medicine. Well, I was going along the road and I said to myself, "God, I feel so miserable, I'd better put on a bright face." And as I did, this man coming towards me caught my eye and we smiled. And do you know, I felt I knew that man, really knew him, I can't describe it. I could have been good friends with him, do you know what I mean? I don't mean to say an intimate friendship, a lovers sort of thing, but something went between us and I think that's what happened with me and Cathy.'

Something happened with me, too, as Sister Paul spoke. Slowly, it began to dawn upon me that Catherine was as strong a character as anyone I could think of. When I knew her still, her potency was directly connected to her psychosis, her crazy mutterings and manic laughter, her disappearances and her occasional but lavish aggression. People were always wondering what she might say or do next. Latterly, however, it seems that she made an enormous impact on everyone she met whilst giving up almost nothing of herself. What force of personality she must have had then, for it to impress itself so tenaciously upon the people she knew whilst she kept it so well-concealed.

'She had that effect on a lot of people,' Sister Paul continued, 'the whole group of us that knew her. You're going to see Betty Wear, aren't you.'

'Yes, that's right.'

'Betty's very good. She's a member of St Vincent de Paul.'

'That's a charity, isn't it?'

'Yes.'

'Is it for homeless people or drug addicts?'

'Any kind. Any kind of people, they come. And Father McKay does so much here, too. It's a very, very poor parish, and we're right in the middle of the drug culture.'

'He's a nice man.'

'Oh, he's a very good man. Excellent. He's human and he's dedicated to the poor. He's a very good preacher, too, and others admire him. I know he was preaching in Wells Cathedral some years ago and the Archbishop of Canterbury, who was Bishop of Bath and Wells at the time, said to a friend of mine who was there, "I do envy the Catholic Church Father McKay." '

'There aren't a lot like him,' I agreed. 'I've met dozens of clergy and people of his quality are exceptional.'

'They are,' said Sister Paul. 'And he wears an awful lot of hats, you know what I mean? At the moment, he's getting a place built for people coming out of prison, a safe home. It will accommodate four men, give them the transition from prison to ordinary life. He's Prison Chaplain as well. I was Prison Chaplain myself, you see, so we have a liaison there.'

Sister Paul stopped.

'But I'm getting off the point,' she said apologetically, and then she sighed.

'When I think about that stretch of road,' she said, and for a moment I was lost, unsure which road she was now on, 'that stretch of road where Cathy walked, I just miss her from it, you know.'

I nodded sympathetically. This was Sister Paul's loss, not mine, of a person she had liked, someone who was a fixture of her daily life.

'She was really lovely, your sister,' said Sister Paul, 'and I think God was very much in her life. The God she believed in which, of course, is the same universal God. You don't believe, you said, when we spoke on the phone.'

'No.'

'No. But you're open to other people's understanding in that way.'

'Of course. You can't close yourself off from what other people believe or you close yourself off from life.'

'Aye,' said Sister Paul. 'So true.'

'I do talk to Catherine sometimes,' I said, 'which is silly really, if I don't believe she's there to hear it. I'm probably doing it for myself. But I've been meeting people who were in her life, and I've been talking to her about it so that she knows that I'm not trying to invade, because I'm not. I'm trying to discover her for myself because it's the only way I'll have anything left to hold on to. It started off, I suppose, as wanting very badly to know that there were people who cared about her. Well, I've learnt that now, and I could actually walk away today, knowing that.'

'That's good,' said Sister Paul.

'I could rest easy now. I know that there were people like you who were part of the fabric of her life. And that's important.'

'You thought she was alone and nobody cared?'

Yes, I thought. I did. Not too often but not infrequently either, before I went to sleep at night, I used to wonder what Catherine was doing. I used to wonder, even more, how she was feeling. Aged fifteen, twenty, twenty-five, thirty, I lay awake in the dark hoping she wasn't lying awake in the dark, hoping she wasn't lonely.

'Well,' I said, 'I worried that there wasn't self-acceptance in her life, and there wasn't calm, and there wasn't friendship or humour, and all the things that were clearly still there. I thought she might have been in such a deteriorated state that she wasn't leaving her flat or speaking to anyone.'

'No,' said Sister Paul, emphatically. 'Every morning, faithfully, she went out. Where she went to I don't know but I'd meet her around ten o'clock in the mornings, and if she lived in St Phillip's it means that wherever she'd been she was coming back. But she was always cheerful and she was always very neat. She was every bit – I wouldn't say a lady but she was every bit a person, and she had dignity. You couldn't determine which sex she was but it didn't matter, it wasn't important. She was a person I liked to meet and I know the others who knew her felt the same. When they heard she was dead there was a genuine shock that somebody had gone out of our lives, and maybe not very much in our lives but nevertheless, a significant part of them. So I think you can feel proud of her.'

'I do, the more I learn about her.'

'Ah yes, do, because she never lost her dignity.'

Sister Paul's face was bright, illuminated by the recollection of my sister. It was good to see Catherine made visible this way, even if it was a Catherine I did not completely recognise.

'The thing about your sister,' she continued, 'was that she

accepted the way she was. I think she found her own identity, as much as she could.'

'Well,' I said, 'that's quite something. We're all seeking to do that, aren't we.'

'Yes. And she was a real person. She wasn't mad. She was eccentric yes, eccentric in the sense that she didn't do things the way other people did them, that was all. And that was fine. Why should we be the same? I was just thinking this morning, and I hadn't thought of it for years: you know how girls are always talking about film stars and everything? Well, when I was a girl I just could not understand why the other girls were going stupid over them, falling in love with this one and falling in love with that one. And I wasn't going to fall in, join them. And I felt glad, you know, when I look back, I felt glad I was myself.'

The telephone rang.

'Oh, bother,' said Sister Paul, hesitating.

'You get it,' I urged her, 'please don't mind me.'

I'm glad you're yourself, too, I thought, as I considered Sister Paul's disappearing form. At what cost, too? I wondered. Had the pursuit of a religious vocation been relatively easy for Sister Paul, or not? Most people think that religious endeavour of her kind means closing a lot of doors – on money, sex, family, a certain sort of individuality. And it does, at least if looked at only in terms of its obvious costs. More common still is the notion that religious life is a form of refuge from the real world, but you get refugees in every walk of life, and there are places to escape to that are far less demanding, psychologically, than convents. Certainly, religious life is a minority choice but to reject a common route in favour of the road less travelled has its own rewards. You don't have to be a nun to recognise that.

How interesting that Catherine should find Sister Paul, this other outlaw in a world full of people trying to belong.

I smiled to myself at the beautiful anarchy of a Roman Catholic nun and my schizophrenic sister sharing formal, Buddhist-style peace on a Bristol street. If anything could persuade me that there is a God, it would be something as asymmetrical as that kind of encounter. Did Catherine recognise the similarities between the two of them, I wonder? Did she recognise that in Sister Paul, with her warmth and her open countenance, there was a fellow dissident? I'm pretty sure she did.

And what did it cost Catherine herself to live as she did, in a very different kind of solitude from Sister Paul? What expenses did she incur along the way? No partner, no children, no job. You could argue that such things would never have been available to her in the first place, that she could not reject that which was not on offer and therefore never know the pain – and the pleasure – of choice. I am not so sure. Catherine was not blind. She could see the world around her. She was aware of what she was not. To reject her own sexuality externally and to contain so much internally must have involved some choice, or at the very least some sense of self-preservation. If it did, then that choice – with all of its intrinsic complications – cannot have been straightforward. Frankly, it won't have come cheap.

Only the day before my visit to Sister Paul, whilst rolling around on the sitting room carpet at home with Clare and waiting for the *Teletubbies* to begin, I had flicked around the TV stations and caught the rear end of a BBC chat show. The presenter was in full flow, concluding an interview with a transsexual with the slick, vulgar expertise of the jeering but seasoned entertainer.

The transsexual in question had been born a woman but was now a man. Accompanying the transsexual on the programme was his daughter who now had, I suppose, a second father instead of a mother.

'Thank you for coming on the programme,' barked the presenter to parent and child, before turning to an elderly woman who had clearly been talking earlier about her son – who had also had a sex-change operation and was now known as her daughter.

'And thank YOU, Mavis,' he leered. 'Will you come back and bring your daughter with you?'

Mavis looked distinctly uncomfortable and fidgeted in her seat.

'We'd like to hear her story and others like it,' he said, turning away from her to face the camera, 'so if YOU know anyone who's transsexual, or you're a transsexual yourself, we'd love to hear from you.'

He turned back to the woman but only partially so, careful to keep the greater percentage of himself camera-wards.

'So we'll see you again, Mavis. WITH your daughter!'

'She's rather shy,' whispered Mavis, looking down at her hands. She appeared to be on the verge of tears. I wanted to wrap her in my arms and remove her from the shabby prurience of cheap daytime television.

'We'll give her a mask!' hollered the presenter, as he turned his perma-tanned face back to camera.

Sister Paul re-entered the room and rescued me from my thoughts.

'You mentioned to me on the phone,' I said to her, 'that you'd had a brother you'd tell me about.'

'Ah, yes,' Sister Paul leaned back and settled herself.

'I had a brother next to me,' she began, 'who was paralysed from birth. And not only that, he couldn't speak. So I've got a tremendous empathy for people who are different.'

'Was he your twin?'

'No, he was nearly two years older than me. And when I was born I think he resented me, and I probably resented him because we were both babies competing for Mum's attention. But he was intelligent, in the sense he knew all that was going on. He could say just two words, "Mum" and "dim", a drink. Thank God the Lord took him because it would have been a hard life for him. As it was, my mother had to put him into a home. We had only a small house at the time, my father lost all his business, he was very fond of drink, and consequently things were very difficult. I used to go to see my brother with my mother, and he'd get a hold of my hair, his fingers were twisted, and he'd get a hold of my hair and he'd pull it. And I'd let him do it because I knew that that gave him pleasure, you know. But when my mother left him he would cry, it was terrible.

'The night my brother died, my mother woke my sister. My sister was sleeping with her. "Maureen," she said, "Joe has died." My mother had felt the curtains by the bed move. In Scotland they used to have those recess beds and she felt the curtain move, and later we found out that he did die at that moment. She said that he came to say goodbye and I'm perfectly certain that he did. She was a Celt, my mother, and the Celts are pretty psychic.'

'How old were you?'

'I was five and I can remember him very well.'

Sister Paul paused and then she leaned in towards me in that particular way I realised that she had, when she wanted to tell you something really important.

'The funny thing was, I was on a retreat once, and this lady was there. And in the course of conversation, before the retreat started, somebody said, "She can interpret dreams." "Oh," I said, "That's interesting, I must ask her," because I had this continual dream with a child in it.

'So she came up to my room and she had a chair there,' Sister Paul pointed to an imaginary chair on the other side of the room, 'and a chair there,' she pointed to a real one by the window, 'and she sat in that chair and I sat in this one.

'And this lady said, "Right, tell me about that dream with the child," and I told her more or less what I've said to you.

'She said to me, "Who do you think the child was?"

'I said, "I think the child in my dream is that brother of mine."

'And she said, "Right. Put your brother in that chair there," Sister Paul pointed to the imaginary chair across the room, "and talk to him."

'I felt such a fool but I said, "Joe, you know, I think you resented me when I came along," and I talked away to him like that.

'Then she made me change places, so that this time I was him talking to me. I did it, and I sobbed over it, you know. It was very, very therapeutic.

'I had one more dream of a child after that. The child and I were going across the road and the child looked up at me and we both laughed and ran across the road together. That was the end. I never dreamed of the child after that. Strange, wasn't it?'

'Yes.'

'So I do believe the dead are in communion with us, you know. And I think you can call on Catherine and talk to her, and just say, "Help me, Cathy, you're my big sister." '

I must have looked a little unsure.

'Yes,' insisted Sister Paul, 'Say, "You're my big sister, come on, we didn't have much chance. Do it for me." You can say that.'

Then she asked, 'Have you ever gone to church at all in your life?'

I thought about the long answer. I was in the church choir when I was nine. I liked the singing and the fifty pence wage each week. Later, I had a very religious boyfriend, so I went to church with him, mis-spent a portion of my glorious youth gazing from church windows at Sunday morning sunshine and wondering why I wasn't still in it, in my trainers, running, as I had been an hour earlier. Eventually, of course, I returned to the Sunday sun – and wind and rain – with full embrace. But if I have an enduring image of being trapped, it is of regarding the weather outside from a place where none can truly penetrate, a place in which I have mistakenly positioned myself, faithless and bored, where nothing grows and I feel myself perishing.

I decided to spare Sister Paul the details.

'Yes,' I said to her, 'but I don't believe now and I didn't then, either.'

'Aye, but you know the Creed, don't you.'

'Yes.'

'In the Creed you say, "I believe in the Holy Catholic Church, the Communion of Saints." Now, the Communion of Saints means that those who are dead and those who are alive are all saints, saints in the making. The Creed is definite about this. God's in his world and so are his saints. And you've got a saint in your family, I'm certain.'

'That's a nice thought,' I said.

'It's true,' said Sister Paul, fixing me with her benevolent stare, and for a moment we sat in silence, saying nothing to one another. I basked in the warmth of the friendship and fortitude that was on offer with nothing in return required, and I thought that for those who believe in God this is probably what prayer feels like, on a good day.

We rose from our chairs simultaneously. Sister Paul was standing closer to me now than most people would care to stand next to someone else but she lacked any embarrassment. Her easy proximity was as unselfconscious as most other things about her.

She held out her arms.

'Give me a cuddle,' she said. 'And let me give you one, for the one I couldn't give Cathy.'

So, in the middle of that dark Victorian sitting-room, we embraced in honour of my sister. I think we embraced, too, in honour of the peculiar ways in which people find one another.

'I'm so glad we've met,' said Sister Paul.

'So am I.'

'She was never neglected, your sister. Not by herself and not by others. She was loved. You must never forget that.'

'Thank you.' I was crying.

Sister Paul wiped a tear from my cheek with her thumb. The gesture was maternal. I dissolved and she held me.

When the moment was right she handed me a tissue from her pocket and looked into my face.

'You tell your mother that your sister's all right,' she said, squeezing my arms tightly. 'She is. Tell your mother she has someone in heaven praying for her.'

'I will.'

I gathered up my bag and we left the room, Sister Paul's keys jingling slightly in her hand. She opened the front door and we stepped out into the drab grey day together.

'I'm glad I knew Cathy,' said Sister Paul, shutting the door behind her and turning the key in the lock. 'You should be very proud. You had a wonderful person in your family.'

Weird Things That Happened, Three: The Mystery of Frank Sinatra

I do not care for Frank Sinatra's music. In fact, I can't even stay in the room with it. My husband, whose skills at mimicry are legendary amongst our friends, regularly sends me fleeing from the kitchen in total recoil simply by singing the opening bars of 'Come Fly With Me'.

According to my trendy friend Sian, who emigrated some years ago to New York, Sinatra's music is classified as 'lounge music' by those who care. Sian once had a boyfriend who came to their relationship bearing hundreds of well-organised vinyl records of lounge music. I asked her how she stood it and she confessed that it had grown on her.

'I've got quite into it,' she assured me, 'hard though that may be to believe.'

'Please don't let me down,' I said. 'You cannot seriously be listening to that stuff.'

When the time came to write about Catherine's flat, I dug out the tape recording of my thoughts that I had made in the week immediately after our visit there, and subsequently put away in a drawer. I'd made the mistake of labelling only the cassette case, and not the cassette tape itself, but as far as I could remember (and I don't altogether trust my memory) I hadn't touched it since.

I sat down at my desk and switched on the tape. Side A was full of Frank Sinatra songs. Frank Sinatra in concert, it appeared, recorded straight from the radio. Side B was blank.

I took out the other tapes I had made, dozens of them. Tape recordings of my own thoughts; tape recordings of conversations with George and Richard McKay and Sister Paul. I opened every one and played the opening and closing few minutes of each side. I spent all morning doing this. I eliminated all possibilities of mix-up and returned to the original tape, utterly baffled but convinced, somehow, that instead of that dreary old crooner, this time I'd hear my own late-night recollections.

Frank Sinatra was still there.

'Catherine?'

There was no answer, and no sound except for the birds outside and the underlying hum of my computer.

'Catherine!' I was firmer this time.

Silence.

'Catherine,' I said, 'if you put Frank Sinatra on my tape, that's a good one. But I've still got Betty Wear to see. I'm going to see her next week. Apart from Jo Fleming, she's the last one, okay? If you're not happy, let me know. But I don't think you're unhappy. I don't think so for a minute. I think you're mucking about.'

I thought of the two most important tape recordings I had messed up in the past: the one I had wiped out by accident, by mistakenly recording over the top of it; the one I had used to record something off the radio, thinking it was blank. That was almost certainly what had happened with Frank Sinatra. I couldn't think how or why, but I

knew in my heart that there had to be a logical explanation.

'Catherine,' I said, my belief in her intervention fading
already, 'I hope it was you.'

The Family Room

It wasn't difficult to find Betty Wear. She was a member of Richard McKay's congregation and he had given me her number.

Though I guessed she was well into her sixties, Betty was still working at a drugs rehabilitation centre in the heart of Bristol.

'If you can meet me at the Centre,' said Betty, 'we can drive back to my house afterwards.'

In Betty's car, I explained to her what I'd been up to. I told her about the dozens of phone calls I had made and the people I had met; Steve Shepherd and Karen Ainsley, Richard McKay and Richard Barrett, George Jefferies and Sister Paul; Louise. I told her all about the nurses at the Bristol Royal Infirmary, and Mr Carpenter. I explained that I was due to see Jo Fleming again soon.

'It sounds as though you've done everything,' said Betty.

'Oh, I haven't,' I said. 'But I'm getting near the end now. I don't think I can do much more.'

'No,' Betty agreed.

'But I look back and still wish I'd done things differently, when Catherine was alive, I mean.'

'Yes,' said Betty. 'I was going to say to you before, that always happens, doesn't it, in any relationship in any family. There are always things you wish you'd done.'

* * *

Over a large pot of tea, Betty explained how she fitted in.
'I used to run what we call the "family room", downstairs
in one of the church day centres,' she told me. 'It was for
mums and young children to come in, and one day, Cathy
came in and I started chatting to her and she asked me all
about the room. She took a great interest in it.'

'And that's how you met her?'

'Yes,' said Betty. 'Because she loved art, what Cathy used
to do was call in and see how it was going in the family
room, because we did a lot of art in there with the children.
Then slowly, she began to come in regularly and we'd talk
about things that we could do with the children through art.
She was really helpful to me. She gave me suggestions and
ideas and she used to bring things in. If she knew where
there was something that would be useful she would fetch
it, I think she even used to go out and buy odd bits and
pieces. She'd appear and say, "Look, can you make use of
this?"'

'What sorts of things?' I asked.

'Materials to go with the ideas,' said Betty. 'Fabric. Card.
Sometimes she would go down to the family room with me
while we did some of the things but very often she would
say, "No no, you go on and do it," and she wouldn't actually stay. But she was really interested.'

Catherine as a kind of informal teaching assistant. That
was a novel notion.

'We started with collages,' said Betty, when I asked what
kind of ideas Catherine had had. 'We were talking about
different ways of doing collages and she showed me how to
use everyday things like rice, grains, things like that. And
specifically, at Christmas-time, she brought me in a lovely
load of glitter that she'd got hold of, to make cards for the
children.'

She brought glitter for the children; specifically, the children of strangers. Yet she never met one of her nephews and nieces. Not once.

'She brought in some lovely silky stuff once,' Betty continued. 'And tracing paper and cellophane. And she was full of suggestions as to how to use them. We made paper flowers, I remember. And although I always had a good supply of crayons, if she came across any she would always think of us. "Look," she'd say, "I found these." '

I recalled some crayons I had found myself, in Catherine's flat. They were in an old red biscuit tin. I had wondered where they had come from originally because they were of such good quality. Bought new, they would have been very expensive. They came from a charity shop, perhaps.

'I would have loved her to have actually stayed and done something with the children,' said Betty, 'but I never got that far with her. I wanted to include her but she wouldn't stay. She used to pop in and if there was somebody around she'd have a few minutes chatting. In fact, it was always the first thing she did when she came in. She would pop in to the family room first, poke her head round the door and say, "Hello, how's things?" And yes, she was a person that kept herself to herself but occasionally we would talk about something.'

'What sort of thing?'

'I would always like to know how her own art was going.'

'And did she tell you?'

Betty thought for a minute.

'Well, she seemed to mind if it wasn't just right,' she replied. 'I know one day she'd done something and she was really uptight that day because it hadn't gone right. And yet I thought it was good.'

Betty indicated the tea pot with her hand, offering a second cup.

I shook my head. 'I'm fine, thanks.'

'So she'd started this painting,' Betty said, 'and brought it in to show me but she wasn't happy with it. Perfection, I think, is what she was looking for. She'd been up all night trying to work it out and she was going to sling it away. "It's not right," she said.'

'What was it of?'

'It was a scenic picture,' Betty replied, 'and what happened to it I don't know. I said to her, "Wait, you never know. Forget it for a bit." But she was convinced it wasn't right. I don't know anything about art but that was the only time I had an insight into what exactly she was like with her own.'

Betty frowned thoughtfully.

'I was very pleased to be able to do that,' she said, in serious tones, 'I was really pleased she felt she could come to me and talk about it. But she was angry about the picture and although she did calm down that's the only time I felt I was included in her art. She was always willing to give me ideas, but with hers it was different and she never mentioned it again. I couldn't bring it up either.'

'She'd done a lot of pictures.'

'Had she?'

'There were thousands in her flat. Really thousands, I'm not exaggerating.'

Betty nodded slowly.

'It seemed to be a way for her to be able to get out some of her feelings,' she said, 'her art.'

'Exactly, yes.'

I asked, 'When you say she was very interested in the family room, was she interested in the children themselves?'

'Yes,' said Betty. 'It was definitely the children she was interested in, wanting more for them, wanting to give them help. I suppose she'd seen people out on the streets with young children, and the families that came in to the Centre were families that were just setting up home. Very often, they'd been on the streets themselves in the past. The women had found they were expecting and then didn't know how to belong to the community, so they would come in and start off with us before they re-integrated.'

In my imagination, I peered into a room full of women and children, each of them lacking something that so many take for granted. Nourishing food, stable relationships, decent housing. Space. Confidence. Trust. I thought of the almost insurmountable problems they brought with them to the family room. Thank heaven, I thought, for people like Betty Wear. And thank heaven for Catherine, too, who knew what wonders might be created with rice and cellophane. She understood the importance of the imagination and the necessity of having an activity. She knew that art was fun and understood its rewards. She recognised how she could help. And she found a place to belong herself, on the periphery of the family room.

I said, 'Did she interact with people much? I've had the feeling from what people have said that she didn't, but it sounds as if as she did with you.'

Betty poured herself another cup of tea.

'Not a lot,' she replied, 'but she did talk to people if they spoke to her. She used to come in for her meals and would stay around during the mealtime but not for very long afterwards. I think about an hour would be the most she would stay and then she would go off again.'

An hour. A whole hour. What a long time that sounded like now. My expectations of Catherine had changed over time. I'd grown so used to tales of the three-minute encounter that to hear of her spending an hour in the company of others was almost shocking.

'I think an hour was quite a long time for Catherine,' I said, aware of the understatement in my voice. 'Did she come and eat here regularly?'

'Fairly regularly,' said Betty. 'The last time I saw Cathy was actually just before Christmas. She came in after she'd been to hospital and found that she had to go in for surgery, and she was very talkative then. That was the last time I saw her. She told me she was ill and we talked about a few things. We talked about what might happen to her when she came out of hospital because she was wanting to know how she could get meals and things, so I explained that there would be a hospital social worker that would help her with things like that.'

'That's right,' I confirmed. 'There was. How did she seem, when she talked?'

Betty paused momentarily.

'You know,' she said, quietly, 'it was the first time I had ever known her talk quite so much. This was why I knew there was a difficulty. I felt that she was really concerned about herself and it was the first time I had noticed that about her. Before, she was always thinking about other people. But I suppose it is a shock when you find out you've got to go in for an operation.'

She frowned once more.

'I honestly didn't realise how serious it was,' she said, almost apologetically, 'because she didn't look any different, she looked the same to me. She hadn't changed at all.'

'But she was concerned about being ill?'

'I think she was more concerned about what was going to happen when she came out of hospital. It wasn't about herself as such, it was the practical things, and I think she wanted to sort that out before she went in.'

Practical things like food and laundry. How often I had heard the words, 'She was always clean, always tidy.' Catherine's concerns made sense, of her personality as well as her fears.

'She cared about her appearance,' I remarked. 'That's the impression I've been given.'

'Oh yes,' said Betty, 'she did. I must say, she had her favourite clothes as well, it's one of the things that always used to make me smile. There was a scarf and a pair of gloves and a pair of trousers that she really loved, and sometimes she needed them for a special occasion, she said. She used to do her own laundry but because we've got a washing machine and dryer at the Centre she would sometimes want to use it. She'd say to me, 'I need it quickly. Can I get this done for tonight?"

'What sort of scarf was it?'

'Red and white.'

'A football scarf?'

Betty nodded.

'She had two or three of them,' I said, wondering how many more than two or three there might have been in Catherine's extraordinary wardrobe. 'I've got them now.'

'Oh, have you? She was always tidily dressed and always had a bag. Have you got the bag?'

'I think I've got it. People have talked about the bag. It was obviously a big feature of hers. Leather?'

'Yes, brown.'

'A shoulder bag.'

'Yes, that's it. Flat-shaped.'

'That's the one. It had all her Rizla papers and tobacco in it.'

'Oh goodness, her roll-ups, yes. Oh, she used to smoke!'

'She certainly did.'

'But I had a No Smoking rule in the playroom and she never broke it. She was always very respectful of these things.' Betty leaned forward once more. 'That's why it's so important to tell you about her interest in the children because she was so obviously very concerned and caring about the children. Even though she wouldn't interact with them she was thinking of them a lot and I thought that was really, really nice. I thought it was wonderful and I valued her. I valued very much what she felt about the room and how it was going.'

I said to Betty, 'You know, hearing all this is quite strange to me. Lovely, but strange. I mean, I've got a baby daughter now, she's nine months old, and all the others in the family have got children. Catherine had eight nephews and nieces when she died and she never met any of them. I'm not sure she even acknowledged their existence. I sent her photos of Clare when she was born but I never heard from Catherine again after that summer. I know now that she was very ill then.'

Betty smiled sympathetically.

She said, 'I really do think this might have been her way of coping with that, maybe. I don't know. But maybe thinking about the children in her family was all she could do, and being involved with our family room here, that was her way she could help. It was the way she could be involved with the children in her family.'

'You mean by loving them at one remove?' I asked, thinking how we all ended up being loved by Catherine at one remove, courtesy of the Royal Mail.

'Yes, I do,' said Betty. 'Maybe.'

'But I would never have expected a family room to be something she was interested in,' I said, still not quite over the shock. 'She couldn't cope with proper family and I simply would never have expected her to want to be near a room like that.'

'I see exactly what you mean,' said Betty. 'But this was something that she could back away from, wasn't it. I mean, it's not close, there are no demands.'

'That's true,' I said. 'And families, even if they're not trying actively to help you but just want to show that they care about you, that can be a demand in itself.'

Betty was silent for a minute, then she said, 'It must have been very hard.'

I shrugged.

'Not for me, really,' I said. 'Much worse for other people in the family. And you get used to it pretty quickly. It was just the way things were.'

'Yes,' said Betty, 'but still.'

'Well,' I said, 'it was always a fine line between letting Cathy know she was cared for and having a proper relationship with her. Because having a proper relationship with someone means occasionally pulling them up short if they hurt you or take advantage – and that certainly happened in the past with Catherine. She'd ring my parents and ask for money but not bother to have a conversation once she'd ascertained that it was forthcoming. She did the same with other people, too. But we were not allowed to make a first move, ever. We were totally on the end of her string: you are if you're on the receiving end of someone with mental illness.'

'Oh, I know,' Betty nodded fervently. 'You are, you are.'

I said, 'A few years ago I wrote to her several times in a row, and I sent her a present and some money for her birthday but heard nothing. And I suddenly lost patience. Even after all those years of knowing full well that she was ill and communication was hard for her, I thought, Well, sod that, she could at least bloody-well write back just once.'

Betty smiled.

'So I wrote her a letter telling her exactly that,' I continued, 'in language I know we were both perfectly comfortable with. She wrote back straightaway telling me how much she had always loved me and how much I, and my letters, meant to her. I couldn't believe it. I hadn't heard from her for so long and then there was this outpouring. I felt terrible, I was filled with remorse. I felt such a heel for being so cross.'

Betty shook her head, sadly.

'That must have been really difficult,' she sympathised.

'It was but I got over it and I don't regret it now. I could have not had a go at her but then I would have been mollycoddling her, wouldn't I, and I don't think she'd have appreciated or respected that. I also think that if you treat someone with kid gloves too much, whether or not they are ill, you're then failing to treat them like an adult or an equal, and that's not right.'

'No,' said Betty, 'that's absolutely right.'

'And of course, when someone's died, you go over all the things you wish you'd done differently. You think, I wish I hadn't blown up at her that time. You think, I wish I'd called on her at home, even though you knew that it was right at the time not to intrude upon her. There's always a selfish bit of you that wishes you had.'

'Yes.'

'And you imagine a scenario in which you'd done so and it would have been okay. But it wouldn't have been. She would have felt caught on the hop.'

'Yes, she would,' said Betty. 'She didn't cope with pressures at all, with demands of any kind, that was quite obvious. Because if I asked her to do anything, like when I was asking her to join in with the children, she backed off very quickly. That's why I never asked her again. Thankfully, it didn't stop her coming back.'

'How long did you know her?'

'Three years.'

'Three years,' I mused out loud. These last three years of her life.

After a while Betty said, 'I don't feel I had a lot to say to you. I'm sorry.'

I shook my head.

Catherine liked children. She wanted them to have a

chance to do something nice. She taught Betty how to make paper flowers and rice collages, so that Betty in turn could teach the children. Catherine provided glitter at Christmas, brought in crayons and card. She ate with other people, would talk to them even. She got Betty to help with her laundry. I thought of the first few things I ever learned about the sister I had not known: that she called herself Stevie and breakfasted on George's sandwiches; that she could still rustle up a Beethoven sonata.

'Oh, you did,' I said. 'You did. You said plenty.'

'Did I?'

'Yes, but everyone says what you did, that they don't have much to say. They don't realise that if there are five people, for example, and they each have a couple of things to tell me, that's ten things. That's ten things I never knew about my sister. That's ten things with which to paint a picture in my mind, ten things for the family archive. They are things to pass on to my daughters about the part of Catherine's life I never knew and never saw.'

'Oh,' said Betty, 'yes, I suppose that's right. Well, I'm glad that even a little bit is helpful.'

'It is,' I said. 'More than you could know.'

Stones Unturned

Amongst the things I found in Catherine's flat was a post card addressed to Stevie Stevenz. It had been posted eighteen months before Catherine's death and was signed, *Your friend, Margaret Taylor*. The card's content was inconsequential. On it, Margaret Taylor expressed pleasure at a recent meeting with Stevie and sent best wishes. The postmark was the local district one, Avon. Although she might have been from elsewhere, I guessed that Margaret Taylor lived in or around Bristol.

I kept the card like a talisman. I had managed to unearth no other personal correspondence at all except the card from me. A few weeks later, I telephoned Directory Enquiries. There were several M. Taylors listed in the Bristol telephone directory and I could be connected to none of them as I had no addresses. Anyway, because listings for married people generally give initials for the male spouse, it was highly likely, unless Margaret Taylor was unmarried, that the M. Taylors in the Bristol phone directory were men.

My husband said, 'Mark will find her for you.'

My husband was doing some work at the time alongside a Corporate Intelligence company rather like Kroll. Mark was a director of the company.

'I can't ask Mark,' I said.

'He won't mind. It'll take him two minutes on a computer.'

'It's spying,' I said, 'it's not legitimate.'

'Firstly,' said my husband, 'it isn't spying. Spying he can do but it's entirely different and it takes slightly longer.

Secondly, it's perfectly legitimate because he will only be accessing information that's publicly available.'

During his coffee break that morning, Andrew emailed Mark. After lunch, I received Mark's reply, which he sent directly to me.

Hope this helps, Mark had written. *Come back to me if you need any further assistance. All the best.*

Attached to the email was a list. It contained the names and addresses of forty-two Margaret Taylors, all of them living in or immediately around Bristol.

'There you are,' said Andrew.

I was horrified.

'I can't do this,' I said.

'Do what?'

'Contact all these people on the off-chance that one of them sent a post card to Stevie two years ago. I can't do it. It's wrong.'

'Why?'

'I'm not sure. It just doesn't feel right. It's intrusion on a massive scale, on her as well as them.'

'Well,' said Andrew, 'you've got the list. You can always use it if you want to.'

But I never did.

Though I did go to Barrow Gurney, in the end. It seemed important at least to know what it looked like, the psychiatric hospital in which Catherine had been resident so many times over nearly twenty years.

It left me cold. The staff were friendly and helpful and the setting spectacular. The buildings were Edwardian with modern additions, set in old, wide-ranging woods of cedar and pine. But I saw nothing of my sister there, except the briefest of glimpses when I met a nursing assistant called Dorothy who had known and liked her.

'And I don't like everyone,' she said, firmly. I believed her. Dorothy was beautiful, with a penetrating gaze and natural authority. That she was now working in a restricted access ward, with patients who were deemed actually or potentially dangerous, did not surprise me.

'But I liked your sister,' said Dorothy. 'She used to make me laugh.'

To reach the ward you had to declare yourself on video through an intercom system, and only then were you allowed to pass through double doors of plated glass.

No knives, blades, metal objects or ligatures allowed beyond this point. No nurse to be left unattended with patients.

It had taken a modicum of persuasion on my part to be allowed to visit Barrow in the first place. Then, having apprised the hospital administrator of my intentions (simply to see where my sister had been), I told a friend of mine who is a psychiatrist in Bristol that I was going there and he kindly offered to accompany me.

We walked the grounds and wards, my friend and I, but the place was not alive for me. I had visited psychiatric hospitals before, and a high-security prison, so some aspects of the environment that might reasonably have shocked me, like its security measures and some of its very sick patients, did not do so. But even so, I was disturbed by glimpses of bodies hunched under thin sheets, by those people too ill, tired or medicated to be up and about in the midday sun. I was saddened by almost everything I saw: the angry graffiti on a bedroom door; the overpopulated smoking room where my smile was met with stares of impenetrable hostility; the beautiful female patient in her thirties who offered to answer any questions, whose relaxed appearance belied her presence there but whose desperate manner did not. These things upset me but not because Barrow was unusually sorry.

Psychiatric hospitals are simply not cheerful places. I was unsettled by the pervasive quiet, as if normal human activity had been suspended and time had stopped, which for most people there it probably had.

There were bright spells, like a patient and nurse absorbed happily in a game of chess, but mostly all I wanted to do on the day I went there was to leave. I had found my sister already. I had enough of her to keep me going.

So I don't know that there was ever a defining moment, although discovering the ease with which I might have contacted forty-two identically-named women came as close as I can think of to being one. And it would not be fair to hold Frank Sinatra responsible. I'd made the decision long before he made his mysterious appearance on the tape that would otherwise have provided me with some useful reminders for my book. Quite when I made the decision, though, I'm not sure. But at some point I decided that there was as much available to me of my sister's life that I should leave untouched as what I had already sought and found.

There were a lot of letters left in Catherine's trail. My parents handed them over to me and I read them all. There were letters that Catherine had written to my parents. There were copies of some of theirs to Catherine, too, and many, many letters about her: letters from psychiatrists, social workers, probation officers and prison governors; letters from the Indian Embassy; letters from concerned but often misinformed outsiders.

There were official letters, loving letters, pleading letters, begging letters; letters offering assistance, letters of sympathy and resignation. There were letters about medical treatment, money and what the future might hold. There were letters written from locations which themselves served to illustrate the nomadic tumult of Catherine's early twenties: letters written from comfortable homes and gardens but also from bedsits, hospitals, beach huts, mountain cabins, hippy communes, and prisons.

There were many crazy letters, some of them horribly amusing, like the one Catherine wrote to the Wantage branch of the National Westminster Bank, requesting that a large sum of money be wired to her in India despite her being newly incarnated and therefore in no need of it.

There were letters from my parents' friends in India, one of whom, Penelope, once talked Catherine out of police custody in Dharamsala and took her to her home in the Himalayas. Then there were the letters from strangers, fellow travellers who had found Catherine in streets at high altitude, shivering and ranting, without her passport.

There were dozens and dozens of letters. Full of colour, they told their own stories. But those stories were not my stories and neither were they mine to re-tell. So when I had read them I put them all back in the files where they are kept, and I returned them.

It could have been something that arose from that uncomfortable meeting with Richard Barrett, inherent in which was the realisation that it was too much to expect other people to reveal my sister to me, plus the sense that I was barking up the wrong tree. It may have had something to do with the fact that no one I met at the cafés she had supposedly frequented had any memory of her. I could have taken my café search further but my encounter with Victor put me off. What the hell, I thought. What the hell if she did come here? Need I know, really? I never found out, either, which café it was that had exhibited her pictures.

There was a hairdressing salon that she visited regularly. Not a barber's shop, which is where she doubtless had her hair cut to within a quarter inch of her head. A hairdressing

salon, the preserve of women. She went there to read magazines and have a cup of tea. Sometimes she was chatty, at
other times not. Occasionally, or so the story goes, she would
just sit quietly neither reading nor talking. I was told this
by Karen Ainsley when I spoke to her on the phone after
our meeting; she had forgotten to mention it at the time. She
explained which of two hairdressing salons it could have
been. I never visited them. By the time I discovered their
potential significance I felt the need to restore the balance
somewhat, to leave Catherine alone in some of the places
she had been and her other acquaintances unaware of my
existence. My desire had always been to find her but I never
wanted to plunder. There are no rules in a situation like the
one I created for myself so I made them up as I went along.
I tried to do only what felt comfortable and decent. I had
things I wished to keep private, too. So I stopped when I
sensed that I had done enough.

It could have been that after meeting the people I did I
had done enough, in both senses. There wasn't going to be
a lot more that anyone could tell me, I was certain. There
might have been one or two more surprises. There would
certainly have been details. Gradually, however, it became
increasingly important to me that I would never know what
they were. For the maintenance of my own probity it was
necessary that some things about my sister's life should
remain as mysterious to me forever as Catherine herself. I
was satisfied, yes, but it was more than that. Enlightenment
comes at a price and it was important that Catherine should
not be the one to pay.

I was also, frankly, just too tired to carry on looking. I
had a baby to care for, a new life to cherish. Five months
after Catherine's death, and less than a year after Clare's
birth, I was pregnant with my second daughter. I was
delighted but exhausted, too, sleep-deprived, nauseous and

after Jane was born, badly depressed for a time. Catherine's Bristol was not the best place for me to be. For more than two years, I stayed away from it. When I returned, it was on paper.

The first thing I found when I went to the file marked *Visits to Bristol* was the following list:

Insomnia
No appetite
Exhausted
Angry for no reason
Don't want to speak to people, hate the phone
Can't think straight
No sense of humour
Can't listen to music
Don't want company but feel lonely all the time
Having terrible nightmares, recurrent. Mostly the children
  are drowning and I
  can't save them
I love my family, it's not them
I can't be depressed, my life is great
I'm just tired

I recognised the writing as my own, and briefly, I was puzzled, but only briefly. The list was one I had made before an appointment with my GP, approximately six months after Jane was born.

'You should have written them down,' said Jo Fleming, of the questions I had wanted to ask her, that dark afternoon in Catherine's flat.

I learned my lesson from my sister's GP and wrote things down thereafter, to help me remember them. I wrote that particular list so I wouldn't forget to tell my own GP what

I was feeling, in order that I might convince her that I was merely sleep-deprived and nothing more.

I was diagnosed immediately with post-natal depression and treated with a moderate course of anti-depressants. Within days I felt much better. Within weeks I was more or less back to normal. But it was over a year before my confidence fully returned, a year during which I experienced new and strange sensations: reticence, non-specific anxiety and shyness.

Reading through that list of what I now understand were symptoms of an illness and not just the usual by-products of maternal exhaustion was a real shock. I could not remember feeling that way but I knew I had. I could not remember all of the things I had experienced, either. I even began to wonder if they were true. My memory of the period during which misery crept up on me so slowly that I did not see it for what it was has become blurred. Certain events or encounters stand out like sharp rocks in a grey sea but I can barely recall the sea itself.

That my list of woes was catalogued amongst my memories of my visits to Bristol was both odd and ironic. It was odd that I had kept the list at all. It was ironic that it ended up in a file where, at a stretch, it could have been mistaken for Catherine's own notes. Except that it could never have been hers. The notes I found in her flat were much more arbitrary and confusing, and she had no children to fear for. But she knew terror-filled nights and so did I. She kept the door shut and so did I. She knew what it was to desire contact while shunning the company and well-meant enquiries of other people. So did I. She did not eat or sleep well. Neither did I. I denied my depression because I didn't recognise it for what it was. At times she denied her illness, even though I suspect she did recognise it, and it frightened her.

We shared more than I thought, my sister and I. Fears and

denials are common currency and few of us avoid them. You don't have to be schizophrenic to experience the horror of a mind gone awry. You don't have to be crazy in the first place in order to lose your grip. It isn't only those mad few for whom the world can seem freakish and bewildering.

It was not a bad thing to be reminded of that fact.

My father had a patient that he looked after for many years, who died after a long illness. As death approached, the patient stipulated that various parts of his or her body should be donated afterwards. (Such is my father's proper discretion that I don't know if the patient was a man or a woman.) My father knew that the eye surgeon at the John Radcliffe Hospital in Oxford was in need of some corneas. In fact, the need was sufficiently urgent that my father telephoned the surgeon almost immediately after the patient's death to say that some corneas could be made available to him. The surgeon asked if my father would be kind enough to remove them straightaway so that he could arrange for them to be collected the following morning. It was the middle of the night.

My father was a GP of the generation that had a fairly comprehensive experience of surgical procedures, so he expected to perform this sort of surgery from time to time. And anyway, or so I am told, removing eyes is not particularly difficult. You just have to watch you don't cut the optic nerves. So, in the small hours, my father removed the eyes of his long-time patient and placed them in a jar of sterile solution in the fridge in the hospital kitchen. His generation of GPs also expected to put body parts in the hospital kitchen fridge alongside the milk and butter without an ensuing public enquiry.

A few hours later the hospital cook, opening the fridge in search of eggs to cook for the patients' breakfasts, came across the eyes. There was hysteria, some vivid cursing of my father and the threat of resignation, which is why I know about the patient, the eyes and the furious cook. This story, with personal details removed but a perfect balance of gore and suspense left untouched, is precisely the kind that my father used to pull out over Sunday lunch in order to induce the delighted thrill of revulsion in his teenage children.

So when people ask me how it is that you can write about a dead sister, I think about a doctor removing the eyes from a corpse once known to him. Regarding his patient in personal terms would not have been helpful to my father when doing what he had to do. Something similar applies to writing about a dead relation. If you are more concerned about how you feel than about conveying how you feel, you will fail completely. Dispassion is oddly possible, when on the job, at least. You cannot indulge yourself in sentiment. And it's not as if anyone is forcing you to do it: unless you're a masochist, you don't choose to write about something you can't cope with.

Curiously, on returning to the papers, tapes and photographs that contained what I had gathered of my sister, I learned that memories proved less potent for me than the workings of my imagination. I realised that the act of writing about things that had happened to me personally de-personalised them somewhat. This is because writing about an experience of your own entails taking a step backwards from it. Objectifying an experience is part of the distillation necessary to turn it into something readable and it tends consequently to render the experience itself more manageable, emotionally speaking. Writing about things that happen to other people has the opposite effect. Bringing to life the experience of someone else demands that you take imaginative steps towards it, which amplifies it.

My father had to remove his patient's eyes with sufficient

care and skill that the corneas were usable. Writing has to be usable too, in the sense that it has to work. I think my father probably enjoyed the challenge and precision of the procedure itself but if enjoyment is too loaded a term, it's fair to suppose that he was totally absorbed whilst remaining emotionally in neutral. The same goes for an average after-noon's writing, whatever the subject matter.

There's a whole other side to this, obviously:

My father in tears, lonely and distraught, publicly rejected by his daughter amongst strangers in a Himalayan town.
Seeing the words, *Lord, this cell is cold* upon the wall of Catherine's room.
Her bed, strewn about with teddy bears, and the curve of her body there still.
Catherine sitting opposite my mother and me in her previous flat, so clearly divided from us by her Michael Jackson montage, her badge collection and her illness.
Locating Catherine's flat, invisible to me for years before, from the window of a train to Penzance as it pulled into Bristol Temple Meads station, and knowing the informa-tion to be useless.

These are things over which I cannot comfortably linger. And it is things like this that represent the sort of emotional wear and tear to which people imagine you are prone when they ask the question: how is it that you can write about your dead sister?

The answer is, you want to. You want to because writing is how you respond to what you see, just as others pick up a camera or a paintbrush. You want to because writing is where you find time and space to ask questions of yourself and others. You want to because you cared about her. You want to because what happened to her is interesting to you.

You want to because other people have relations who are lost and you hope to start a conversation, even if it is one in which you may take no active part. You don't do it because no one else is doing it or because you think you owe someone something. You do it for yourself.

But you have to learn to be content with what you've got. A post-mortem search is fine, an attempt at resuscitation futile. It goes for the death of anyone, close to you or not, sane or not. In order to release yourself from your own sense of loss you have to accept that there will be no more of them. You have to understand that while you may seek more, even discover more, they are finished. However you come to know someone after their death may change you but it cannot change them. Resurrection is impossible.

So it is important that certain things remain undone. It was necessary to me to stop looking for Catherine while there was still more I might have found. That stones are left unturned is the bargain we make with the dead.

PART THREE: BEGINNING

A Journey's End

Jo Fleming came to Catherine's funeral wearing a brightly-coloured Indian scarf because it had been one that Catherine had especially liked. Afterwards, she left in a haze of silent tears.

How wrong I had been to doubt her.

The surgery was not easy to find but Jo's directions to it were good. Strict navigation was required for a route through residential streets of shabby housing punctuated at the corners by petrol stations, newsagents and small grocery stores. Billboards advertised computers, cars and mortgages that most people living in this part of the city would have too little money to buy.

The surgery car park was a modest space, nicely bordered with mature shrubs. No need for a car park fit to accommodate the bulging company cars of the fat south-east, or even the fatter parts of Bristol. Here, most people probably walked to see the doctor, or caught the bus.

The building itself had a lot of glass. Not the grey place of my ruminations, it was luminous with sunshine borrowed in advance from another season. As if the month of May held all of June in reserve and had exploded under the pressure, the day was fierce with premature heat.

I entered through automatic doors. There were no patients around. It was an afternoon for GPs to do home visits or paperwork and Jo had put aside her time for me.

We sat in her consulting room with mugs of tea. Jo's young

sons, in school uniforms, beamed at us from photographs lined up along the shelf above her desk. A very pretty cardboard train ran alongside them. One of Catherine's pictures of Tibet adorned another, higher shelf.

'How many children do you have?' I asked.

'Four boys,' said Jo, glancing up at the photographs. 'They're quite a bit older than those photographs now, though. The eldest is just about to start university. The next one down is starting Sixth Form this summer.'

It didn't look possible, that this youthful woman should be the mother of nearly grown men.

I recalled my first meeting with Jo at Catherine's flat, her hands in her pockets, her head low, her voice quiet. I remembered my own body cold and tight in defence. Any wariness that might have existed between us had been dissolved by the letters and emails we had exchanged in the four intervening months. Jo's greeting to me now was warm and open.

All the same, even after the funeral I had been nervous of approaching Jo, this loyal confidante of Catherine's. However, there were so many questions gnawing at me that I felt compelled to do so. One of them concerned me personally almost as much as my sister. Yet when I first wrote to Jo, even at her invitation, I was frightened of rejection, of being told politely to go away. I was worried that she might regard herself, quite understandably, as chief custodian of Catherine's later memory and concerned that any stance she might take could prejudice her against me. I was afraid of seeking help and finding myself cast right back into the shadows by the one person whom I believed might shed some last light upon the mystery of my older sister.

Most of these fears were now alleviated but I outlined them to Jo nevertheless, in the dense late-May sunshine of her consulting room. A small part of me was still waiting to be told to put away my tape recorder and go home without the final piece of my sister.

'Well,' said Jo, calmly and quite deliberately, 'Cathy's dead, and when people die there are sometimes people left behind with their own needs. I don't see any problem with that. I'm certainly allowed to talk to you if that's what you mean. It would be different if she were alive, obviously.'

'Obviously. But it's still very nice of you.'

Jo smiled.

'It's not a problem,' she said.

'I wrote down some questions this time,' I said, 'only a couple of them, anyway. But then I left them at home. I never write questions down, I don't like doing it. Even when writing my books, I've never done it. It turns conversations into interviews and that's not what I do.'

We chatted. Jo had liked Catherine a lot, it was clear. I wondered what it was about my sister that had engendered so much obvious respect and affection. What had Jo's many years of conversations with Catherine consisted of? It was so long since I'd had one with Catherine myself that it was hard to imagine.

'I miss Cathy,' Jo said, after a short while.

I was grateful for such candour.

'What do you miss?'

'Her humour,' said Jo. 'She had a great sense of humour. And her dignity. She was a very proud person, in a good way.'

'Was she easy to talk to?'

'Mostly. Not always. Sometimes you just had to listen, that was all she wanted.'

I could remember listening, not understanding. I could also remember losing patience on the phone a couple of times, a long time ago, I must have been around fourteen or fifteen. Unable to cope with Catherine's manic ramblings

I made excuses to terminate the conversations. I had teenage
friends in the room, giggling. 'I've got to go,' I'd said, though
I hadn't.

'Would you have called Cathy a classic schizophrenic?' I
asked Jo.

Jo called Catherine Cathy.

Cathy. Cath. Stevie. It was all the same to me now.

She nodded in response to my question.

'Yeah,' she said. 'She did fit the bill, in that she would hear
messages and voices that were not there, and she would have
her own pathways of thought or speech that were directed by
things that weren't available to anyone else. Her suppositions,
the things that she based her day-to-day actions on, were
things that were unreal or things that nobody else could see,
so she was having injections to try and minimise all that. And
basically, when she kept up to date with her injections then
she was more like normal, and when she didn't keep up with
them she became almost frightened and sometimes aggressive
– not physically aggressive but angry about things. She had
tremendous feelings of persecution, of paranoia.'

Clearly, some things had not changed all that much for
Catherine. She was always convinced of dangerous betrayals
and fanciful plots, of voices that told her to do things, of
military surveillance of her home. I thought about the crazy
phone calls I had tried to draw to a close and I wondered
now, as I had then, why it is that so many schizophrenics
are fixated upon the Secret Services and the Messiah. I could
remember it so well, her paranoia, her belief in the omnipres-
ence of MI5, her certainty that people were after her. This
sense of persecution was not restricted only to herself. It
extended to the supposed control of whole nations,
depending what was in the news at the time, although the
very real plight of the Tibetan people almost always featured,
albeit in a surreal way.

'She talked about Tibet to a lot of people,' I said. 'A lot of people who knew her didn't have very straightforward conversations with her but she would talk to them about Tibet. Did she talk to you about it?'

'Yes,' said Jo. 'She came across as having a very great love for Tibetan people but it left her with nightmares. I don't know what happened and what didn't happen there. Do you?'

'No, I don't. I do know she never went to Tibet itself. She certainly went to Dharamsala, in India. The whole thing's pretty confused.'

'Right,' said Jo. 'But she was very clear that even if certain things didn't happen, as far as she was concerned they did.'

'Exactly,' I agreed.

'She talked about being shut in a cell in the dark,' said Jo, 'and hearing people scream about her. She said she listened to the torture that was going on around her and so she was unable to sleep in the dark after that.'

So that was what lay behind her fear of the dark. Recollections of torture. I remembered all of the lamps and candles in Catherine's room.

I asked Jo, 'You mean she slept with the light on?'

'Yes, I think so, and I think she stayed up at night a lot. That's the impression I got.'

'Me, too. She used to do that when she was still at home with all of us. And somebody else told me she played a lot of music at night. I think she was asked to turn it down a few times.'

I wondered if Catherine's fears had increased or decreased over the years, or remained about the same. I certainly recollect her being nocturnal. She paddled around our parents' house at night when she was younger, muttering and laughing, or sat up playing her recorder and singing Buddhist chants. She put the household on edge. Yet it's easy to understand the lengths to which a person might go in order to avoid the peculiar horrors of a nightmare, should she be certain that one awaited her.

I'd had one myself the night before coming to visit Jo. I dreamed I was ordering coffins for everyone in my family, including Clare, from a cheerful, bearded wood merchant in a large sawdust-filled workshop. I was doing so, I told him, 'because you never know when everyone's going to die'. He was delighted with my order. 'Oh, that's great,' he said, pulling out a pencil from behind his ear and scribbling some calculations on a length of oak board, 'because I can get you a special offer on the wood for that number of people.' I had seen *Newsnight* the evening before the dream, in which the Foreign Secretary was being questioned about the pros and cons of the Euro. In my dream the Foreign Secretary appeared (sporting long dreadlocks, I've no idea why) and questioned me about the economic viability of bulk-buying coffins.

I don't think I had an answer for him. I woke up in a hot sweat and clutched my husband in relief before rousing Clare from sweet, damp sleep so that I could hold her close in love and gratitude – my warm, alive baby.

I asked Jo, 'Did Catherine's schizophrenic symptoms get worse or stay the same in the time that you knew her?'

'I think schizophrenic people tend to burn out,' Jo replied, 'that's the term psychiatrists often use. And when they do, they become more in line with normal living and normal attitudes. Certainly she was much more likely to go over the top when she was younger, when I first knew her.'

She picked up a biro from her desk and began to roll it between her fingers.

'I don't know,' she continued. 'She hadn't had any contact with psychiatric services for quite a while, through her choice, basically. She was offered psychiatric back-up in the form of a Community Psychiatric Nurse, and psychiatrists offered to see to her on a regular basis but she turned them down. It's usual for the CPNs to be doing the injections and monitoring people but Cathy refused it. So in an ideal world, she perhaps would have been managed better, medically, but she wasn't exhibiting such difficult symptoms or finding life so hard to cope with that we had to. I mean, she wasn't so bad that it was necessary to do this legally, to admit her to hospital under a Section. It was a very long time since she'd been admitted, though she admitted herself voluntarily, not that long before she died.'

'I see.'

'I mean, she still had her notions, if you like.'

Jo paused for a moment.

'Her flat,' she began.

I waited while Jo twiddled her biro.

She said, 'I know I had been to visit her at home, years ago. The flat she was in then, I remember it being ordered, crowded with her collections but things were ordered. But when I went to her flat, the last visit I made to her before she died— '

'When was that?'

'It was about a week or so before she died, to be honest. When I went then I could still see the semblance of this order but she'd lost the ability to look after – well, you saw the flat. Now, whether that was her physical illness, I don't know. Obviously, by the time she'd had her breast cancer diagnosed she had secondaries.'

So Jo had not known about the flat, not until the very end. She hadn't let Catherine moulder there sick and untended on the grounds that it was the right thing to do, or worse, the politically correct thing to do.

I felt relieved. I told her so.

'Right,' said Jo. 'No, that was only the third time I'd ever been there.'

'Yeah, well, I'm pretty glad about that,' I said, 'because I remember on that day we first met, when I said to you about the flat, "This is an unhappy place," you replied, "Well, I don't know," and I instantly thought, Am I missing something? I felt so foolish at that moment.'

'I'm sorry.'

'It's not your fault,' I reassured her.

'I took a lot of things from the flat the day I saw you,' I continued. 'I took the polar bears and some of her paintings and some watches, other bits and pieces. I took some of her writing because I wanted to see if I could find any sense anywhere. I took some football scarves. It was you who told me they were important.'

'Yes?'

'Yes,' I said. 'And I was grateful because I didn't know what the hell to do in there. I also photographed the flat. I told Cathy I was doing it, I talked to her while I was doing it, explained why, but what amazed me is that the photographs were not what I expected at all. When they came out they were so vivid, so bright. It was a really disgusting day that day, do you remember, and there were no lights, so I used the flash on the camera and all these colours have come up so brightly in the pictures.'

Jo nodded. She was listening intently.

'And when my husband and I left I thought I'd never go back there.'

She nodded again.

'But there was still a horrible gap to the funeral, the gap was long, ten days or so. A couple of days before the funeral I thought, We've got to get all the pictures off the wall that are still there because if she put them there it was because they were special. So I rang Steve, the caretaker, and he was kind, he took them all down for us.'

A picture of the walls that morning flashed before me.

Stripped of Catherine's paintings, the writing on them fully revealed, they were all the more stark.

mean   with   his   fists

'The morning of the funeral,' I said, 'my husband and I went to collect the paintings. It was a beautiful day, do you remember, cold and sunny, really clear. In the garden at my parents' house there's a large stream and it has steep banks running alongside it. Catherine had planted some of those banks with snowdrops when she was a teenager. I only discovered that after she died. My mother told me. So I picked a load of snowdrops early that morning and I put them in the flat for her. I put them on her bed.'

Jo was looking very sober.

'Going back there then,' I said, 'it was so calm, so light, the flat felt quite different. The day that you and I met there I was absolutely convinced she was there too because I've never in my life felt such a strong presence, not a hostile presence but an extremely wary one. But when I went back the second time, she'd gone. She'd absolutely vanished. The flat was still full of her stuff but empty of her.

'For a couple of weeks after that, I grappled with that flat all over again. I grappled with the right of people to live the way they wish. I had real difficulty with the idea that you might have visited her often and possibly done nothing practical to make her living conditions better. But also I thought that if you had known, you probably would have made all the suggestions you could have done and they had probably been rejected. And I was quite wrong about it all because you hadn't been there much at all.'

'No,' said Jo. 'I hadn't.'

We sat silently for a while, drinking tea.

'I don't know,' Jo said at last. 'It's very hard to imagine what she might have been thinking or going through at that time.'

I said, 'For a long time, when she was alive, I wondered whether she missed us. But now I have to accept that I don't think she did. I've almost stopped asking myself questions about why she was or wasn't very much in touch with us because it's pointless. And also, Catherine had only done a more extreme version of what a lot of people do. Even though it's common for schizophrenics to distance themselves from family, and from people in general, you don't have to be schizophrenic to need to do that in order to be your own person.'

'No,' said Jo, 'you don't.'

'So, like I say, I've stopped asking questions about that because I just don't think they're relevant. And also, frankly, I'm sure she didn't give that much thought to it herself, so why should I? I mean, I don't think she was sitting at home thinking, Shall I be in touch? Are they thinking of me?'

'I'm sure she didn't,' said Jo, with feeling. 'Yeah, I would be almost a hundred per cent certain that she didn't. I mean, I certainly think she thought about the family and she had good memories. She talked a lot about you, she thought the world of you.'

I thought, But she didn't know me any more than I knew her.

Jo said, 'But I don't think she sat there pining or worrying.'

'No. We did the worrying.'

'And she certainly gave the impression,' said Jo, 'that she took each day as it came, so while she had plans, and they were big plans, they were almost on a shelf. You know, they were something she was going to do one day, perhaps.'

'Plans for her own life?'

'Yes. And grand schemes that would sort things out for the whole of the nation. She had plans for the UK and the world.'

I smiled.

'Who doesn't?'

'True,' said Jo, 'but hers were very clear. She held very strong opinions about various things, particularly animals and particularly Tibet. Those were her major concerns.'

I thought of all the stuffed toy animals in Catherine's flat and her donations to the WSPCA and Guide Dogs For The Blind. I thought of all the paintings of Tibetan monks, some of them angry or weeping behind Chinese chains and bars.

'What do you think?' I asked Jo. 'How much was that flat a really painful place to be or a safe place to be, for Catherine?'

'I think it was both,' Jo replied, quietly. 'I think she felt very, very vulnerable at the end because she felt unable to cope there. I could see that she was struggling before she went into hospital, when she was at the beginning of the last bit of her illness. I know she was scared and I know that's why she didn't go for the appointments with the Consultant that I first made for her. Although I don't think that if she had gone things would have been any different, to be honest.'

'No,' I said. I was thinking how obdurate cancer is, and inscrutable; how often it gets the better of us.

'I don't know how long it was before she had noticed the breast lump,' said Jo, 'and how much she was trying to ignore it because wanting to deny things can be true of anybody. She came to me with the breast lump, I said it needed sorting out and I tried to be firm without being scary, which is quite hard, even though I was quite convinced that she had cancer.'

'The other thing,' Jo said, 'is that GPs don't get notified of hospital appointments, the hospital contacts the patient directly, so I didn't know how things were progressing for a little while. But then I had a letter from the hospital saying she hadn't been for two appointments and asking what was happening. So I went to try and find her at that point and couldn't. In the end, I caught her outside her flat and she said she was scared about the lump but she allowed me to bring her back to the surgery and re-examine her, and she allowed me to make another appointment for her. She wasn't just scared of whether she had cancer or not because she actually asked me if I thought it was cancer and I said that's what I was worried about. She was scared of being laughed at and ridiculed because she didn't feel or look like a normal woman of her age.'

My mother had said more than once, 'Poor Catherine. I only hope someone told her that men get breast cancer, too.'

'So I promised her,' Jo went on, 'that I would contact the clinic and tell them that she had these concerns, and I tried to reassure her that of course they wouldn't laugh because even men have breast cancer, it's not solely down to women.'

'I'm very glad you said that,' I told Jo.

'Oh, I did,' said Jo. 'And then I think the lung secondaries were beginning to flare up because she did start coming in and catching me more often. I think it was about a week later, when I was doing a Saturday morning surgery and she was here, that I was able to admit her to hospital because she had chest pain. She was asking for admission then because she really wasn't feeling very well, and of course in the old days I could have admitted her much sooner and said, "This is what we're concerned about. Can you sort it out?" '

'But you can't do that now?'

'No, you can't. You have to have a specific reason for being admitted and it has to be for the limited reason only. That's what it's like in Bristol and I would say it's probably true of anywhere. But I was able to admit her at that point, on the Saturday, and I explained to the hospital the concerns she had.'

I pictured Catherine being admitted to hospital, shown to a bed, given directions to the shower and the smoke room. I tried to imagine what she must have looked like at that point. I tried to picture the cancer itself, unsuccessfully: I didn't know what cancer looked like.

'Which side was it, just out of interest?'

'Right side.'

'I just wondered,' I said, not knowing why.

It is commonly said of women, by men, that they want to know all the details. It is commonly said by women that men confuse details with basic information. A friend once rang us to announce the birth of his new baby and my husband put down the phone not only without its name but its sex.

'But he must have told you,' I said, bursting with frustration.

'Yeah, I think he did,' my husband replied, casually, 'but we were talking about other things, too. I've forgotten. I'm pretty sure it's a boy.'

'You're pretty sure?!'

'Well, I can't remember the details,' he protested, 'it's a baby. Do you want to ring him back?'

'I think it was the right side,' said Jo. 'I can have a look if you want me to because it will still be in my computer. In our computer network there's some glitch in the software so nobody disappears. Even if you die, you carry on getting older.'

'A virtual ageing process,' I remarked. 'That's a bit Orwellian. What happens to people's notes when they die?'

'All the written notes go back to the Health Authority and they keep them for a certain length of time,' said Jo, and I imagined a giant basement room filled with row upon row of A4 manila files reaching as far as the eye could see, like crosses in a military cemetery.

'You know,' she said, 'if you'd wanted me to have them here today, I could have organised it.'

'Oh no, it's fine. I just wondered.'

'We're not allowed to throw anything away and we don't take things off the computer when people die, they stay there.'

I looked at the computer on Jo's desk.

'So there she is, getting older.'

Jo looked at it, too.

'Yes, curiously. I don't think she'd be very happy about it.'

'No,' I agreed. 'She probably wouldn't. If anything was going to induce paranoia, it would be that.'

We had reached a natural hiatus in the conversation. There would be no more avoiding the most important question of all. 'You'll get what you're given,' I say to my daughters when they're making too much fuss about precisely which sausage or potato they want on their plates. My mother used to say it to me. Well, I was about to get what I was given. I hoped I had enough courage to accept it.

Jo rolled the biro between her fingers. I played with a paper clip that was lying on the desk.

It was swelteringly hot.

'When Clare was born last summer,' I began, 'our house was just awash with cards and flowers. When Catherine died, most people who knew she'd died, they didn't mention her, they didn't write, they didn't respond as they might to a different sort of death. Obviously there were exceptions and you can say to yourself of the others, "Well, people don't know what to say," but I think that's a lame excuse. I was really shocked by the lack of response or by the flippant nature of some of the reactions I had – no, not the flippant nature, the callous nature. People saying it's a mercy, saying it must be a relief. People saying, "At least it was cancer and not something worse." "Worse?" I'd say, "Well, the cancer did the trick." '

'Absolutely,' said Jo. She looked pretty shocked.

'The more it happened, the more angry I was. It got to the point where I thought, Damn it, how dare they, everyone has value. I mean, Cathy had value to you. She had value to all the people who knew her, and what I've learnt since coming to meet people down here is that wherever she went, she got respect. People really respected her for who she was.'

'Yes,' said Jo, fervently, 'absolutely.'

'Which is partly why I want to write this book. To have her dismissed so roundly, so easily, felt so wrong. And yet I know there were times in the past when I did it myself to an extent. I know there were times when it was easier to think of her as lost to me completely because trying to maintain a relationship with so many obstacles in its way was difficult.'

Jo nodded.

'So I started writing at first just for myself, simply because she was my sister. I felt I had been left with so little of her that whatever still existed I should record it before it, too, just vanished into thin air. I wanted to know what she'd been doing with herself all those years. I wanted to know where she'd been. And it gave me something to do, I suppose, when I felt impotent and miserable, though I was miserable on behalf of other people, really, much more than for myself. But now, the writing has begun to develop into something beyond the private because I feel that people don't understand what a life like Catherine's means. Not just other people: I don't fully understand it myself. There are so many questions for me now, questions that I've never considered before about the value and quality of an individual life, and they arose partly because so many people made instant judgements about the quality of Catherine's life, even people who had never even met her. So many people thought she was a waste. So many people clearly thought us better off without her.'

'Those are all very good reasons to be writing,' said Jo.

'Maybe,' I replied. 'Maybe not.'

I hovered for a moment on the brink of my question.

'But I've wanted to ask you for a long time,' I said, finally. 'And I have to ask you straight. Do you think Cathy would mind? Would she mind me writing this book? Because I think you're the only person who'd have a genuine sense of that. Plus, I believe you'll tell me the truth.'

Jo looked at me straight in the eye. She would tell me the truth.

'I don't think,' she said carefully, 'that Cathy would even presume to tell you what you could write about how you felt, right? So I don't think there'd be any concerns there and I don't think you should have any. She would have no worries about that. She might laugh at some of the things you felt because – well, she just would. But she was the one person I know who would respect people for what they felt. You know, she never made judgements. She didn't judge anybody and that's what she asked for in return. If she got that, if you just accepted her for who she was, and respected her for what she did, even though you may not have chosen to do it yourself, then she was happy. That was what she wanted. So I don't think she would mind at all you writing what you felt, or how it's affected you. You can't write about how it affected her because you don't know.'

'No, absolutely not. One can only suppose.'

'I think the other thing to say to you,' continued Jo, 'is that whenever anybody dies there will always be somebody who will say the wrong thing. If your father had died, somebody would say, "Well, he had a good innings."'

'Yes, I know they would.'

'And if a baby had died, somebody would say, "Well, you can always have another one." People will try to say things that make them feel better without always thinking about what it's doing to the person.'

'I know.'

'They're trying, of course, to be comforting.'

'Yes,' I agreed, 'which is why I haven't been cross with anybody, although I've felt it.'

'Well, you should feel it,' Jo insisted, 'because I think people should think about what they're saying before they say it. I mean, it wasn't a mercy for Cathy to die. She wasn't relieved that she was dying of breast cancer at all. She had life to live and didn't want it to stop.'

Jo sighed but not wearily, there was some passion in it.

'She knew she was dying at the end,' she said, sadly, 'I'm sure of it. And she didn't want to die on her own. She was really scared about being left in that flat, the day I re-admitted her.'

'Re-admitted her?'

'Yes. She'd been sent home from the hospital when they felt there was no more that could be done for her.'

'Had she?'

'Yes.'

'I didn't realise that. I knew some plans were made for her to go home, but I didn't realise that she had done. Was she happy about that?'

'No. She kept on talking about how plans were being made around her. She said, "Everyone's got plans. Everyone can make plans to make it okay but it's not okay." You know, "Your plans aren't helping. The plans won't work." She was very fixed on the way that we were planning everything so that she could stay at home and she didn't want to stay at home, she wanted to be with other people.'

Catherine the recluse. Catherine who rarely allowed people

in to her home and wouldn't volunteer her name. Catherine who denied her family and walked the city streets alone. In the end, even she baulked at a solitary death.

Yet I was confused. Louise, the social worker I had met, who had made all the arrangements for Catherine to return to her flat, said that Catherine was determined to be at home. I explained this to Jo.

'They wanted her to go home,' said Jo, 'the hospital, that is, because it's felt that people should have the right to die at home where their things are and they're comfortable and in their own space.'

'Of course,' I agreed, 'but why did they want her to go home if she didn't want to?'

'Because I think they have this mind-set that the place to be is at home. "We can't do any more for you. You're going to need to be at home. We can arrange everything so that it works for you and home is the best place to be because you're in your own space." And we go along with that because we believe people have a right to do that. You know, people are usually more comfortable at home.'

I said, 'But a lot of people have got comfortable homes, and people in those homes. Catherine didn't.'

'Yes, that's right. And also, the arrangements that had been made had been made without going to the flat. They had been made over the phone to people. You know, "Go and clean the flat for her, then she can move back into it." Well, somebody had obviously got as far as the front room, they'd cleaned the bathroom and the hallway, and stopped because they didn't know what to do after that.'

'Yes, well. You wouldn't, would you.'

'Quite,' said Jo. 'But they hadn't reported back to the hospital. Cathy had been given a mobile phone but she didn't know how to use it. They showed her but she wasn't up to it. Somebody else thought they'd organise all her medication in packs so she could just take out the amount that she needed at any one time. But they didn't show her how to open the box, so when she did try to open it – she had a lot of fluid in her hands and she wasn't very dextrous – the whole thing had just fallen apart, so all her tablets were muddled up.'

Oh God. Those broken packets of medicine I found on the floor by her bed. When I thought of Catherine struggling to open them with fumbling, swollen fingers a sharp pain went through me, the pain of wanting to help my sister and knowing that I never could, never had been able to.

'She'd been given food,' Jo continued. 'But her fridge didn't work, so the cheese and the milk would go off.'

I thought, Please don't let this account get any worse.

'So everything was there,' said Jo. 'The thought processes were there. You know, "We'll sort this problem out and that problem." But it hadn't been done from the facts of her flat. So she got home and the doorbell didn't seem to work, so she couldn't let anyone in, even the District Nurses couldn't get in.'

Trapped inside again. Not even by illness this time, just by a doorbell. There was help outside and she wouldn't have known.

'So it was thought through,' said Jo, 'but not enough. And maybe she did express desires to go home.'

'She might have,' I said, 'at some point. The social worker was quite adamant that she had. I'm sure she was telling the truth.'

And I was sure, too. I could now see how all this had happened. I understood that the institutional will was there to aid my sister. Louise seemed to be a diligent woman and I could appreciate that the mechanisms for helping Catherine, and indeed anybody else returning home to die, were all in place. In fact, they were quite impressive. Their fault lay in the fact that they were thorough but not foolproof, efficient but not all-encompassing. Yet how could they be, really? How could a general plan for the domestic care of the terminally ill take into account a life like Catherine's, a home like hers? It could and should do but it is easy to see why it doesn't. That she suffered made me bitterly sad but that she was failed by a system was no reason to be angry. At least there was a system. At least people tried.

'Having got home, she then would have had problems,' Jo said.

'I know Louise saw the flat once,' I said. 'She said that Catherine hadn't wanted her to but she had seen it once. But I don't think that was post-cleaners.'

Jo laughed and said, 'It's irrelevant really, isn't it.'

'Oh, it is irrelevant, yes, in terms of what you might see. But it's not in terms of whether decisions were made before or after seeing the flat. Louise said it was the most personal flat she'd ever been in to. She said she could see why, if that flat was your space, you'd want to go back into it. But then Catherine clearly didn't want to be there when she was cold and— '

'Yes,' Jo interjected, quite fiercely, 'and she was cold there. She was uncomfortable. She wanted to be back in hospital. It was quite clear,' she said, firmly, 'that it was inappropriate to send Cathy home.'

Underneath, I felt, Jo was still seething about it.

I played with the paper clip some more, turned it over with the tips of my fingers.

'How did she express that distress?' I mumbled, not sure that I really wanted to know.

Jo replied, 'She didn't ask to be re-admitted, she didn't tell me how bad she was feeling, but she very clearly communicated that this wasn't what she wanted now. I suppose the nicest thing would have been for her to go into a hospice where it's a bit more home-like but they don't have the beds available just at the drop of a hat, unfortunately.'

'I was told by Louise there were plans for her to go to one.'

'Yes, there was a plan,' said Jo, 'but I don't think she lived long enough. I'm just glad she wasn't on the Medical Ward with the nurses fussing around her.'

I knew exactly what Jo meant but thought, nonetheless, how unfussy were the nurses that I had met.

I said, 'They told me at the BRI that they'd put her on her own because she wanted that. I think they treated her very well on that ward.'

'Yes, well,' said Jo, 'I think there, as everywhere, she was liked. People adored her. The only people who had difficulty with her were the ones who like to categorise people first and then deal with them afterwards. And I think if you're doing oncology you can't be that sort of person.'

'No,' I agreed. 'And they nursed her as a man as well, and that's – it's wrong to say it's remarkable but I think it's really good. Really good. It's not, perhaps, what you might expect. And I'm sure that must have helped her. I spoke briefly once to a woman on the phone, called Nicola, who was a volunteer attached to the Midland Road Methodist Centre. Nicola knew her for the last three years of her life, I'm not quite sure in what capacity. She said to me that she was always struck by Cathy's jewellery. She said there was something actually very feminine about her even though she liked to be Stevie.'

Jo nodded. Clearly the sentiment struck a chord with her.

'No one else has said that at all,' I added.

Jo said, 'She had what people think of as very feminine qualities. She was very aware of people who were less fortunate than herself, people with difficulties. She had very big concerns, social concerns. I remember one time she came in and was beside herself because she was worrying about the dogs that homeless people have. She said that if you're homeless you shouldn't have a dog. She said it was very wrong, that it was irresponsible.'

'Dogs were her thing,' I said. 'She loved them.'

'They can be easier than people,' said Jo.

'How long had she been Stevie?' I asked. 'Do you know? Did she suddenly decide she was Stevie, as far as you knew?'

'As far as I was concerned, she was always Cathy.'

'I know she was for you,' I said, and it occurred to me that remaining Cathy for Jo was a measure not only of the longevity of Catherine's relationship with her doctor – eighteen years – but also of her absolute trust in her. 'But she wasn't for everyone.'

'No,' agreed Jo. 'And it came as a surprise to me when the people in the Treatment Room called her Stevie. So I don't know. As far as Maria, the practice nurse, is concerned, she's always been Stevie, and I don't really know when that happened.'

'Well, from what you said to me about the set-up here when I arrived today, it's at least eight years, isn't it, since Maria first knew her.'

Jo did some mental calculations.

'Yes,' she agreed. 'And Cathy always dressed in a manly fashion. But only once did she ever say anything about her name to me, and it was some muttering about how people assume you're a man and then somebody calls you "Cathy". I said, "Well, change your name on our computer, there's no problem, so nobody calls you 'Cathy' at all." But in fact, she said no, she didn't want that. So she was always Cathy to me.'

Jo nodded and the affirmation was for herself rather than for me.

'Yeah,' she repeated, 'she was always Cathy to me.'

I said, 'It sounds like she wanted to be both. Because when I've thought about this, one of the things that's occurred to me is that she was perhaps only doing what an awful lot of people do when they play out roles. You know, they go to the office and they're someone different, or they come to the practice and they're Dr Fleming, then when they go home, they're Mum. She didn't have a job and she didn't have a family, so she didn't have an environment in which to play out roles, and maybe we all need to do that and she was simply responding to a need. I don't know. I'm not suggesting it's all wonderfully straightforward but I don't think it's as odd as some people do. I know that some people I've spoken to think it's very bizarre, and I don't really.'

'No,' said Jo. 'I think the dressing as a boy, and calling herself Stevie, was protection in a way. I don't think it was a sexual statement in that she was looking for women.'

'Oh no,' I agreed, 'no, definitely not.'

'In fact,' said Jo, 'I always got the impression she was quite innocent about it.'

'Yes,' I said. 'I think she might have been. I'm not sure she was ever looking for sexual relationships, actually. She never had a lot of boyfriends. The last one we knew about bit the dust when she was about twenty-one. But I do know, from what I've been told, and from what I remember of her, that she didn't ever seem comfortable being female. She never seemed to feel at home in herself. My mother said she used to cry if she had to wear dresses.'

I remembered one of many summer afternoons spent idling with my friend Sue when we were both about sixteen. We were reading *Jackie* magazine and looking through my family's photo albums.

'Who's that?' asked Sue, peering hard at a picture of Catherine.

I could see exactly whom she meant. I played for time.

'Who?' I asked, leaning over her shoulder.

'This person here,' she said, and she giggled. 'He looks really weird.'

'Oh,' I said, 'I'm not sure. Hey, have you seen this one?' and I turned the page.

'Do you think being Stevie and Cathy was difficult for her?' I asked Jo.

'I don't think she found it difficult being Stevie. She didn't like it when female things intruded, you know, like periods.'

'No. I remember you telling me about that at her flat. That you'd given her something to stop them.'

'That's right,' said Jo. 'I think she had found a way of being that suited her and she was comfortable with.'

'I think so, too, mostly.'

I told Jo about Catherine's notebooks from the flat, containing all the medical writing.

'Did she ever talk to you about that?' I asked.

'No,' said Jo. 'Having said that, from time to time she'd come in and say, "I want to talk to you about something," and she'd sit down and ask me a physiological question about the way the body worked, and did I think "the men" could take her theory further? And as long as I obviously listened to her and told her what I could about what I knew, she was happy. In fact, when I think about it, those sorts of conversations tended to be the initiating conversations I had with her over the last few years.'

'The things she wrote about over and over were diseases of the blood,' I told Jo. 'That seemed to be her main interest.'

'Well, she got into thalassaemia, I seem to remember. That and sickle-cell disease.'

I said, 'I was kind of surprised that there was nothing written in her notebooks about mental illness and nothing about cancers. Maybe they were too close to the bone. There's quite a lot about HIV, which I don't think is necessarily that significant, except that it's an illness that predominantly affects the sorts of people that Cathy would probably come across day-to-day more readily than most of us.'

'Maybe,' said Jo, 'But I think she also got interested in things that were in the news.'

'That would make sense,' I said, 'because there was also a lot of stuff about the Russian submarine that sank with all its sailors on board.'

'Right,' Jo said. 'And she got very concerned when Harold Shipman was shown up. She came in and told me in confidence that she was worried about a certain patient that she felt one of the other doctors was killing off.'

'Oh, your poor colleague! How unjust.'

Jo laughed roundly and put her hands on her knees.

'Would you like me to show you round the surgery?' she asked.

'Yes, I'd love that.'

We emerged into the significantly greater heat of the waiting area. It looked now, with its empty chairs and neatly stacked magazines, as if it were waiting itself, for patients. Posters on the wall explained the dangers of smoking, the hazards of obesity and the symptoms of diabetes. Notices were written in Hindi and Bengali as well as in English.

'Cathy never liked waiting in here,' said Jo. 'She couldn't handle all the other people. Mostly she waited outside, round the back, and had a cigarette. But if I knew she was here and waiting I'd always try to see her straight away.'

Although I tried to I couldn't envisage Catherine standing and jittering in here: this space held nothing of her for me. Yet leaning against a wall with a Rizla roll-up out the back, that I could imagine. I could see her as she leaned forward to inhale the first breath of tobacco, forehead furrowed beneath her impossibly short fringe, hands cupped around the tiny cigarette and a lighter, her fingers skinny and yellow.

I could see the canvas shoulder bag and the wide watch-band around her wrist. I could see a bulky jacket, mannish boots, her thin legs in dark jeans. I remembered the chunky, tarnished silver rings on her fingers. I fancied I could very nearly smell her.

Jo led me across the waiting room and down a corridor to a door that opened into a bright, white room of some considerable size. She put her head around the door. A woman in a white coat was inside.

'Hello, Maria,' said Jo. 'Are we disturbing you?'

'No, not at all,' said Maria. 'Come on in.'

We were in the Treatment Room, the place where Catherine was given her monthly injections because she refused to receive them at home from the Community Psychiatric Nurses.

'This is Cathy Loudon's sister, Mary. You remember Cathy,' she said, adding, 'Stevie.'

'Oh gosh, yes.' She smiled broadly and stared at me.

'You did say she was coming,' she said to Jo, and she looked at me. 'How lovely to meet you,' she said.

'And you,' I agreed, extending my hand, which she shook. I looked around the room, trying to picture Catherine in it.

'So it was you who gave Cathy her injections?' I asked. I didn't have the energy to start referring to her as Stevie. It was just too hot, for one thing.

Maria laughed.

'When I could,' she said.

'How do you mean?'

'When she didn't run away,' replied Maria, drily.

'What, literally?' I asked.

'Oh yes,' said Maria. 'She used to go and hide in the car park behind the bushes. You could hear her laughing. I think she wanted to be found. She could be very naughty some-times.' I got the feeling from Maria's robust tone that she had had more than a few words with my sister.

Maria said, 'It was quite a game for her, sometimes, I think.'

'That figures,' I said, remembering – or at least remembering being told – how Catherine had managed in her teens and early twenties simultaneously to exasperate our parents and paralyse them with worry each time she disappeared. Catherine in the bushes, all over again. I thought of her lurking in the shrubs outside the hotel in Delhi while our father waited for her inside, desolate and wretched, preparing to leave the country without her, unaware how close to him she still was.

'Wasn't it, Jo?' said Maria. 'Like a game for her.'

Jo smiled in recollection.

'It was,' she nodded.

'But we usually got her in here between us, didn't we,' said Maria. 'I've gone and found her in the street before now, and you,' she said to Jo, 'would get in the car if necessary and go and find her, wouldn't you.'

'Sometimes, yes,' Jo said, mildly.

'You down here for a while?' Maria asked me.

'No, just the day. I've got a baby at home and I only came down to meet Jo, anyway.'

Maria was scrutinising me with the intense interest of someone trying to match the new and unexpected face in front of them with one from the past.

'I can definitely see a resemblance,' she said. 'Can't you, Jo?'

Jo nodded, non-committally I thought.

'You're quite a bit younger,' said Maria.

'Thirteen years,' I said.

'Right,' said Maria. She smiled some more and shook her head. 'Oh, we do miss Stevie, don't we.'

Jo nodded.

'She was a great character,' continued Maria. 'Infuriating at times, mind you, but we got on just fine, we had our understanding. And it's definitely not the same without her. I'm very sorry about what happened to her.'

'You knew her since you came here, didn't you,' said Jo.

'That's right,' said Maria. 'She was a fixture.'

'And you knew her as Stevie,' I checked. 'Is that right?'

'That's right,' said Maria. 'Stevie. I never knew her as Cathy, she wouldn't let me call her that.'

She looked at me and said, almost more to herself than to me, 'So you're her sister. Well, I am pleased to meet you, I can't tell you how pleased.'

Jo and I returned to her consulting room.

I said, 'I'm so grateful to you.'

'It's nothing,' said Jo.

'It's not nothing to me,' I said.

I could have said more. I could have told Jo how generous and unassuming I thought she was, how intelligent and kind. I could have told her that quite apart from being a good GP, I thought she was a wonderful friend to Catherine and I was grateful. 'You took her as she came,' I wanted to say. 'You let her be. That's what a friend does.'

But I didn't say it.

I said, instead, 'You were amazing to Catherine. You've been really good to me.'

She shrugged but I could tell she was pleased, in a quiet sort of way.

'If there's anything else I can do,' she said, 'anything at all, just let me know. I'm happy to help.'

'That's really kind. I'm sure there won't be.'

'Well, if there is,' she said. 'And good luck with the book. You must definitely write it. You mustn't worry about that.'

'Thank you,' I said. 'I won't.'

I gathered up my stuff and took a quick, last look around the room. I had a pretty strong hunch that I'd see it again one day. I looked at Jo's boys once more, smiling from the shelf, human beings so vital and fresh, poised on the right side of innocence. Then I glanced one more time at the cardboard train. It had been made by a person with some talent. Jo had probably picked it up at a craft fair, or on holiday somewhere.

'I like your train,' I remarked.

'It's nice, isn't it,' said Jo. 'Catherine made that train for me when one of the boys was born. I really like it, too. It's been up there for years.'

Now

What to take, what to leave?

My daughters are playing in the garden of our home in Oxfordshire. I am sitting not far from them, on a bench on the terrace overlooking the stream. The ducks in the stream are quacking noisily. The sun is shining. My husband is due home in an hour.

At my feet are four plastic crates. They contain the things I took from Catherine's flat. Her pictures are not here. They are in a cupboard in our house in Wales. Sometimes, when I go in to it, I see the blurred edge of a tiger's face through translucent plastic.

I do not know what to do with all her things. It has taken me four years to dig out these crates. I've been dreading them but not for the sorts of reasons you might expect, not because the thought of going through them is painful. I've been dreading them in the way you might dread clearing out the attic or doing a tax return. Also, they are smothered in dust so thick that it's almost adhesive. Tackling these particular relics is going to be a filthy job. It is why I'm doing it outdoors and not inside.

I open one of the crates and the smell overwhelms me. Four years later and here is Catherine's flat in all its dark, damp pungency, released into Oxfordshire's fresh spring air. I sit, stunned by the strength of the evocation, transported elsewhere. This, truly, is time-travel.

Inside the first crate, on top of everything else, rests a solitary cassette tape that has escaped from the box in which the rest of the tapes are packed. *Leeds Parish Church Christmas Carols*. It is almost certainly the one belonging to the Methodist Centre, that Richard Barrett mentioned Catherine borrowing. A piece of folded paper has become stuck to the back of the case. I peel it off and unfold it. It is a letter to Catherine from the former hostage, Terry Waite, clearly written in response to one from her. I remember finding it at the flat. In it, he thanks Catherine for her paintings and recommends that she contacts a friend of his. The friend is a psychiatrist in Sussex. Terry Waite, when he was released from captivity, must have attracted a fair number of odd correspondents.

From the crate, I pull out a large red tin that once contained biscuits. On the lid Catherine has taped a tiger's face cut out from a greetings card. I remember the tin from the flat. It contains dozens of long, wax crayons, the ones I thought too expensive for Catherine to have bought new. Jane spies it straightaway and joins me. Her face lights up, expectantly.

'Is that for us, Mummy?'

'Yes, darling. Let me just give it a wipe.'

She hangs her face over the edge of the tin and peers inside.

'There are crayons inside,' she cries, thrilled. 'Clare, we've got crayons!'

Clare looks up from what she is doing.

'Did you buy them, Mummy?' she enquires.

'No,' I say. 'They belonged to my big sister, Catherine. Your aunt.'

'Is that Catherine whose polar bears I've got?' asks Clare.

'Yes, that's right.'

I had washed those polar bears in the washing-machine,

twice on a hot cycle, and gratifyingly, they turned polar white. I love the sight of them now in my daughters' beds: Catherine's inheritance.

Polar bears really get to me, Catherine had written to me once, inside a greetings card with a photograph of one on the front: *So clean*! She always used the phrase 'get to me' in a positive, not negative, way.

I empty the tiger tin and wipe it inside and out. I blow hard on the crayons and put them back in the tin.

'They're very dusty, Mummy,' Jane observes. 'You have to blow them.'

'Well, they're a bit less so now,' I say. 'See, most of the dust has gone.'

'Not all of it, though,' says Jane, solemnly.

'No, darling, not all of it. It would be pretty hard to get rid of it all.'

Jane takes the tin and begins placing the crayons neatly, in twos and threes, on the plastic plates with which she is playing.

'They're toast fingers,' she announces.

The things I really want are Catherine's notebooks. I found several at the flat, partially visible on the surface of that sea of objects. In the subterranean depths were doubtless others. I looked through them at the flat and once again a few weeks afterwards. I remember thinking how little they had to say about Catherine's life, except that she was ill. When I found them I was hoping for the sorts of occasional musings that make sense of a person and in part they did, but only inasmuch as they confirmed the psychosis I already knew about. Otherwise, they left me nonplussed.

I open the notebook in my lap. Just as I occasionally still look for Catherine's missing initials on my parents' kitchen wall I wonder if now, after all this time, there may be some change. I wonder if now the notebooks might read a little differently.

They do not. I leaf through the first four pages of one. On the first page is a detailed description of the sinking of the Russian submarine, the *Kursk*, in the year 2000. It looks as if it has been adapted from a newspaper report. On the second is an impassioned plea for Tibetan freedom. The third page is a shock. Incitements to commit violence are scrawled in angry, jagged lines across the centre. On the fourth page is a detailed biro drawing of a bottle of Boots Fragrance Free Hand Cream.

I had been hoping for something more definitive than that.

I look up at the girls. They are absorbed in play.

I carry on reading.

There are pages and pages of the medical notes I had described to Jo, mostly on AIDS, Blackwater fever and leukaemia. There are diagrams of blood cells and drawings of platelets. Arrows pointing towards them denote the direction of the incoming attacks from viruses or bacteria that they are about to sustain.

And between the medical notes there are poems about Tibet and quasi-political statements interspersed with the odd cartoon or self-portrait, and other notes on various miscellaneous subjects:

Oct 3 Tues approx 7.30
Stapleton Road
Broken suspension car approx 1 yr old
White Sierra
Left hand side leak

Marigold extract mask
A soothing mask for fine and delicate skins

Changing seats evolutionary territory
As in cafes and buses
See Darwin
Artificial face mask

I shake my head. What a fool I am. I had been hoping for something more definitive from Catherine's writing? More definitive of what? If evidence were needed as to my sister's disjointed sense of reality it is here, in black and blue. These notebooks of hers are as definitive an expression of a broken mind as I could ask for.

Reading her notebooks is not like reading her letters. For all their strangeness, her letters usually have a date and a context, and some sort of narrative continuity. What is most confounding of all about the notebooks is not the arbitrariness of the pain and violence that they contain nor even their baffling juxtapositions. It is their lack of context. It is impossible to know what relationship, if any, exists between anything written on one page and the next of any of her notebooks. There is no mechanism for deducing what proximity may imply. It is impossible to know what Catherine was thinking when she wrote them, or what she was feeling, or even when they were written although in some cases references to what were clearly current events, like the sinking of the Russian submarine, the *Kursk*, provide clues.

The *Kursk* sank in the Barents Sea less than six months before Catherine died and she seems to have been pretty obsessed with it. In addition to what look like the adapted newspaper reports of its troubles she has written of her own misgivings. 'Oh yeah?' she has written, beneath a Russian government spokesman's explanation for the sinking. She was convinced the accident that befell the vessel was no accident and the tardiness of the Russian government's rescue mission due not to incompetence but intentional malfeasance. She was actually not alone in feeling this way. Plenty of people cast suspicion on the official reasons for both the sinking of the submarine and the subsequent failure of a group of international divers to reach its stricken sailors until days later. Folded into the notebook is an envelope addressed to a Russian civil servant. No doubt Catherine intended to express her concerns to him.

You don't have to be schizophrenic to be a conspiracy theorist. However, Catherine was badly burdened with serious delusions common to the schizophrenic. Her imagination was rife with plots and subterfuge, so the fate of the *Kursk* will only have confirmed to her what she already suspected, that spies are everywhere and sanctioned murders commonplace. In all this, I begin to see how vulnerable Catherine was in ways that are not immediately obvious. I see how easily, in certain circumstances, a psychotic woman's writing could be her undoing. Had Catherine been in the wrong place at the wrong time – on the perimeter of some kind of genuine violence, for example – what succour her most fanciful scribbling would have provided to anyone wishing to implicate her. What better to propagate the theory of the lunatic than damnation by the lunatic's own hand? Holding these tattered pages of Catherine's, I see more clearly than ever the consummate damage done to her by schizophrenia. I also understand that sanity is a far better form of defence against so many of life's injustices than I had ever previously considered.

I realise I have been hoping for the impossible. I think back to that afternoon at her flat, and how urgently I excavated those piles of rubble in search of something alive and healthy that I could recognise. Her notebooks I thought would be just that. I believed they might hold the key to it all, to the mystery of the person incarcerated in her psychosis. In one sense, they do: I sought a prisoner's diary and I found several. But they contain little evidence of any life lived outside that prison. I see now that I was seeking a refutation of Catherine's psychosis, not confirmation of it. I realise it wasn't something definitive I was after. I wanted an indication that beneath Catherine's exterior was a sane person, trapped and able to express as much.

Further on in the notebook Catherine has made a list of hymns:

Old Rugged Cross
Jerusalem
At The End of The Day Just Kneel and Pray
Abide With Me
How Great Thou Art

Did she want these at her funeral, I wonder?

With my daughters close by I pause, then read on.

There are so many pages and their contents are more alarming than almost anything I have ever seen. The more I read, the more fervently I understand that they are not the way to get to know Catherine, or Steve. The best way to get to know my sister was the way I chose, by walking her streets and meeting her friends. So what of these notebooks? Still the best and sanest of her thoughts to which I have access are her letters to me with their jokes, their snippets of news and their affirmation of love. But these tattered writing pads, with evidence only of Catherine's brokenness, what good are they? Reading them is like being trapped inside someone else's mind while they visit hell. So grotesque and fantastical are the delusions that they tell you nothing about the person who is beleaguered by them. They reveal only a human being at her most vulnerable and least controlled.

I realise now that I will never know what Catherine was thinking on a good day. I will never know what she felt when she walked down a street, ate a meal or painted a picture. I will never know her from the inside out, only from the outside in. But at least now I know my sister in a way I never did before. Now, I have some sense of her life and something damaged has been partly restored. Years ago, she was lost to me, a relative stranger. Now I have found her again, still recognisably the sister I loved.

And today, here I sit, encircled by some of her possessions. But people do not belong to one another and I have never wished – or tried – to take possession of Catherine herself. And that is why I cannot read these notebooks again. They are not mine and it is not okay for me to have them. It is an accident of my own making that they are in my possession and now is the time to return them. I believe Catherine would have liked Clare and Jane to have her teddies and crayons; she would have been pleased to observe her Hawaiian-style garland of flowers hanging from Clare's bedroom curtain rail and her little wooden horse on Janey's shelf. But I do not believe she would want anyone to see her vision of dystopia, a vision suffused with distress, fear, violence and confusion. I do not believe Catherine would ever have wished to share it, not even with me now, in the sun, more than four years after her death.

I snap shut the notebook in my lap.

I think of the words written by the philosopher, Wittgenstein, words I have never read but which my husband quotes occasionally: *That of which we cannot speak, we must pass over in silence.*

I put the notebook on a pile with the others, and I place the pile away from the plastic crates.

When my husband returns, I will ask him to make a small bonfire.

Barely a day has passed since Catherine died that I haven't thought about her. Now, it's rather nice. She wanders in and out of my mind lazily, like a cat moving from sun to shade and back again on a hot afternoon.

In the early days it was different. At the swimming pool each day Catherine accompanied me lap after lap, keeping pace with me. Two months dead, three months dead, four months dead, six months dead. I could keep her at bay in the house but in the water she was obstinately present.

From a friend's swimming pool, one summer afternoon, I observed Clare playing on the grass with my husband, her white-blonde curls a halo around her head, and I saw Catherine. I saw her as she was in a photograph aged about four, a small girl with fuzzy blonde hair back-lit by the afternoon sun, ignorant of the pain and isolation that was to follow. I swam to the side of the pool and leaned my head on my arms. It gets you sideways, grief.

It got me sideways for a good year or more after her death. Asleep, Catherine populated my dreams. Awake, she could be found in unexpected places: one of her watches in a broom cupboard; forgotten paintings in a blanket chest; three letters amongst a batch from someone else. After her death, reminders of her physical presence assumed a significance that they had never done during her life.

In my dreams she assumed many versions of herself. In one that I had immediately after her death, she was walking away down the lane outside my house, waving behind her. 'Bye,' she called, across her shoulder. 'See ya.' In another, I came across her living on a Bristol street. She was very defensive and afraid that I might mock her but I persuaded her to come with me. I took her to a café for breakfast and then on a bus ride through Bristol. She was twitchy in exactly the way that I remembered her. She couldn't keep still, she was rolling cigarettes, giggling to herself and unable to maintain eye contact.

Then there was the dream of the life that she did not have. On a gorgeous sunny day I went to visit her. I knew she was already dead but she was living – in some kind of afterlife – in a very beautiful, plain flat in a Cathedral Close somewhere. The cathedral was enormous, looming up behind the flat. The flat itself had white-washed wood floors and was spare and clear. She was sitting in an armchair with a peppermint-striped cover, reading a book, and when I arrived she was very calm and delighted to see me. She had a visitor, too. A portly man breezed into the flat, greeted her, and breezed out again.

After we had talked inside, Catherine and I sat outside at a table on a lawn. Her home was the only domestic building for miles. She was totally surrounded by the cathedral, a cathedral school, and lots of ecclesiastical buildings and lawns. There was not a single other person around.

I had that dream shortly after going to see her body in the mortuary, her body from which there emanated such extraordinary vibrancy and tranquillity. And although everything in me that is rational resists such notions, I have come to see that dream as a heavenly dream, a dream of Catherine in her present, peaceful incarnation.

Yet when I think of my sister now it is not in a heavenly state. It is in many places and situations, some of which I can only imagine. But among my own memories the clearest are of those magical nights, those nights when she would seek me out and take me to her bed. I remember the psychedelic painting on her bedroom door of the woman with tendrils for hair, and the mobile that she had made from some twisted driftwood picked up on a Hebridean beach. It hung from the ceiling high above her bed, moving in gentle spirals in otherwise imperceptible breezes. I think back to those nights quite often and what I remember is my sister's affection. I remember being cuddled, tickled, told stories and asked questions. I remember secrets being imparted, not secrets involving MI5 or the Dalai Lama, just ordinary ones like: 'The Penguin biscuits are hidden on the top right hand shelf of the larder and if you get the stool from the kitchen you'll be able to reach them.'

So I remember her as she also was. I remember her sane.

Our lives are predicated upon basic cultural certainties. Among the most critical of these certainties is that life should be lived within particular parameters and that human beings possess, if you like, a default setting of normality from which any significant deviation may be regarded as a cause for concern, or worse. That our ideas of normal behaviour are so firmly established allows many people genuinely to wonder what a life is for if it is lived on the border of sanity. It allows them to uphold the belief that life is only worth living or, more serious still, that you are only worth your life as long as you are reasonably happy, well and rational.

For many people, it is important to decide where others belong because it is the only way they know where they are themselves. But it can be very chilly on the edge of their reason. As that old boyfriend sought to comfort me, 'Darling, I'm so sorry, but you know what? Some people are made for this world, some people aren't.' Well, Catherine was made for this world, so damn you (is what I should have said). She was part of this world: dust, ashes, flesh. But attitude is powerful and people like my sister are banished to obscurity as soon as they begin seriously to deviate. Never mind the curtains closing around the coffin, that is only the last of it. Much more effective is eradication of the cursed by the ignorance of the spared.

There is no emotional vocabulary for expressing how deep is the void left by people like Catherine. There is no easy way of convincing the unconvinced that her life mattered, especially as that life was terrorised by mental illness, filled with extreme sexual confusion and cut short by cancer. To many people, such a life makes so little sense that death is the only comprehensible part.

Well, not to me. I see Catherine and I see something comprehensible. I see someone who died in the thick of her life, with plans for the future. I see a woman who did not lack friends, ever, for wherever she went, there were people that liked her, looked out for her. There was always someone she could call upon, and if she wanted company or assistance she sought and found it. She had a home and an occupation. She was prolific. She engaged with the world outside. She created a routine for herself within which she could operate comfortably and she stuck to it. Her sense of humour and her courage never deserted her.

Catherine sustained a lot of damage in her lifetime and caused some, too, and there will always be a way of describing her life as a waste, her existence as a tragedy. There will always be those who see her and others like her as blighted and flawed, although I will never understand the criteria by which they judge. After all, what is a good life, well-lived, and who says so? Catherine simply did what most of us do. She worked out how to live within her limits and she lived as fully as she could. I have tried to explain my sister to myself but she needs no justification. She was her own accomplishment.

Disappearances

I did keep one page from Catherine's notebooks, and this is what was written on it.

Disappearances

(Soul as smoky or seen)

The soul will be seen as smoky or actually there

1. *Set aside clean room for family.*
2. *Cushion for each person with person's name clearly written in front of it. Carefully remember who sits where.*
3. *Light one candle, one incense stick. Offer tea and food.*
4. *Hold photograph or possession of each person, then sit quietly in a moment's prayer.*
5. *Talk & talk & talk to them for half an hour. Some will answer. Some will not be able to.*
6. *Then say, 'goodbye till next time', smiling.*

Blow the candle out & stop incense sticks. This gives them safe return to heaven till the next time.

Author's Note and Acknowledgements

I should like to thank my entire family, but especially my much-loved siblings, for their love and support; most of all, for respectfully leaving me alone to write my rather solitary story, and not expecting to be part of it – as I could never speak for them. However, my parents, Jean and Irvine Loudon, and my husband, Andrew St George, make some fleeting appearances throughout the book, and I am grateful to them for allowing me to refer to them. Very special thanks to my father for the use of his diary.

For giving me permission, in the course of writing this book, to refer to my meetings and conversations with them, I should like to thank wholeheartedly the following people, without whose unwavering support and contributions I could not have written the book at all:

Karen Ainsley, Richard Barrett, Keith Carpenter, Jo Fleming, George Jefferies, Valerie Jefferies, Richard McKay, Sister Paul SSJ, Steve Shepherd, Betty Wear; the nursing staff at the Bristol Royal Infirmary Oncology Centre; and the staff at Barrow Gurney Psychiatric Hospital, Bristol.

In the Chapter entitled *Dreams and Nightmares* I have made liberal use of the written work of Ming Tsuang and Stephen

Faraone, whose book, *Schizophrenia, The Facts* (OUP, 1997), proved invaluable to me while writing my own. Although many of the clinical definitions of schizophrenic symptoms that are described in this chapter are widely agreed upon within the psychiatric community, some specific wording used in my chapter is adapted from Tsuang and Faraone's book, with gratitude.

Those seeking advice and information about schizophrenia can contact the charity SANE at 1st Floor, Cityside House, 40 Adler St, London, E1 1EE, or telephone 020 7375 1002. SANELINE, a telephone helpline for sufferers and those close to them, is 0845 767 8000 (calls charged at local rates). To volunteer to work for SANE or SANELINE email volunteer@sane.org.uk or telephone the London office.

This book was an accident of fate, grief and fascination, and I never planned nor expected to write it. When I began to, two years after my sister's death, I never imagined that it would elicit such frank and generous responses from readers. I always hoped that sharing my own story might possibly help others to cope, understand or simply consider. Indeed, it was the principal reason for writing the book. So I should like to thank all those people who have written to me, and who continue to write, since the book's first UK and overseas publications. It has been a great privilege to hear your stories, and heartening to be a small part of a global conversation.

DEAR LAURA

Letters from a Mother to her Daughter

June Hird & Laura Hird

A daughter's tribute to her vibrant and beloved mother, this book is dedicated to anyone who has ever had to let go of the thing they love most.

June Hird – thwarted actress, insatiable reader and self-confessed romantic – is her daughter's staunchest supporter and harshest critic. When Laura leaves home, June is heartbroken, and keeps in touch with a lively stream of letters. They are full of advice (some good, some bad), scolding and encouragement, gossip about friends and family, hopes for her daughter and regrets about her own life. Deeply moving, funny and wise, these letters are as inspiring as they are entertaining.

"It will make you smile and it will make you cry. A brilliant tribute to the power of love and one woman's passion for life." John King

£7.99

ISBN 978 1 84195 899 6

GARDEN HOPPING

A Memoir of Adoption

Jonathan Rendall

Jonathan Rendall was adopted in the 1960s, when it was easy. People could just pick out the children they wanted, right down to the colour of their hair. But what of the children themselves? Here is one man's search for kith and kin, written with such humour and unabashed honesty that by the end you'll feel like part of the family.

"It's brilliant and it's touching and by the time you've reached the end, you know exactly what the title means." Tom Wolfe

£9.99

978 1 84195 596 4 (13-digit ISBN); 1 84195 596 5 (10-digit ISBN)

IN MY SKIN

Kate Holden

"I made money I'd never imagined and I wore velvet dresses and shone in lamplight. I walked tall in crowds, knowing myself to be desired. I told people I was a prostitute, and smiled as I said it, and dared them to turn their gaze . . . The smile that I give when I talk about it now is, I can feel, nostalgic, provocative. A brightness comes into my eyes. And I'm told, a hard look too."

In My Skin describes an extraordinary journey through an often-hidden world of heroin and prostitution. Kate's story is one of survival and resourcefulness, and an unflinching look at the consequences of addiction.

"Quite simply in a class of its own . . . the work of a stunningly talented writer." Joanna Briscoe, *Guardian*

£6.99

ISBN 978 1 84195 931 3

www.canongate.net